VIROLOGY MONOGRAPHS

DIE VIRUSFORSCHUNG IN EINZELDARSTELLUNGEN

CONTINUING / FORTFÜHRUNG VON
HANDBOOK OF VIRUS RESEARCH
HANDBUCH DER VIRUSFORSCHUNG
FOUNDED BY / BEGRÜNDET VON
R. DOERR

EDITED BY / HERAUSGEGEBEN VON

S. GARD · C. HALLAUER · K. F. MEYER

1

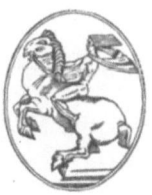

1968

SPRINGER-VERLAG

WIEN · NEW YORK

ECHOVIRUSES

BY

H. A. WENNER AND A. M. BEHBEHANI

REOVIRUSES

BY

L. ROSEN

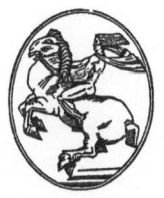

1968

SPRINGER-VERLAG

WIEN · NEW YORK

ISBN-13:978-3-7091-8208-6   e-ISBN-13:978-3-7091-8206-2
DOI: 10.1007/978-3-7091-8206-2

Softcover reprint of the hardcover 1st edition   1968
Library of Congress Catalog Card Number 67-30771

Printer: Steyrermühl, A-1061 Wien, Austria
Title No. 8328

ECHO Viruses

By

H. A. Wenner and A. M. Behbehani

Section for Virus Research, Department of Pediatrics
University of Kansas, School of Medicine
Kansas City, Kansas, U.S.A.

With 4 Figures

Table of Contents

For information:

The increasing number of symposia and reviews provide information on current problems and progress in virus research. Such discussions and "stock-taking" are not only stimulating, but are of great value. In addition, however, a comprehensive and detailed presentation of proven and established results is indispensable and essential.

The editors of "Virology Monographs" aim to publish separate monographic treatments of individual virus species. Particularly emphasized will be the presentation of important findings and their critical evaluation giving extensive consideration and reference to available literature. This new monograph series will continue in the same tradition as the "Handbuch der Virusforschung", also publishing general topics on the technique and problems of virus research, thus maintaining the encyclopedic character of a reference work.

To assure rapid publication, individual manuscripts will be published in form of separate monographs. Smaller contributions will be combined with others to form one monograph volume.

In order to perpetuate the tradition of the Handbook, these single issues will be gathered into Handbook volumes with an index as soon as a sufficient number of issues is reached. In such cases the publisher will inform booksellers and other interested parties that these Handbook volumes are gatherings of monographs already published earlier on.

Zur Information:

Über aktuelle Probleme und Fortschritte der Virusforschung orientieren — in stetig zunehmender Anzahl — Symposien und Übersichtsreferate. Für den Virusforscher sind derartige Diskussionen und „Standortbestimmungen" zweifellos anregend und von großem Wert. Ebenso erwünscht, ja geradezu unentbehrlich ist jedoch auch die Darstellung gesicherter Befunde. Die Herausgeber des Handbuches möchten daher den Schwerpunkt der kommenden Bände auf die monographische Abhandlung einzelner Virusarten legen, wobei die kritische Bewertung der Befunde und die weitgehende Berücksichtigung der Literatur ein besonderes Anliegen sein sollen. In diesem Sinne wird das Handbuch vornehmlich den Charakter eines Nachschlagewerkes erhalten. Der Tradition des Handbuches entsprechend sollen aber auch in Zukunft allgemeine Fragen der Technik und Problematik der Virusforschung Aufnahme finden.

Im Interesse einer raschen Veröffentlichung werden künftighin eingereichte Manuskripte selbständig als Monographienbände ausgegeben; Beiträge geringeren Umfanges werden mit ebensolchen zu einem Band gekoppelt.

Um die Tradition des Handbuches fortzusetzen, werden diese Einzelveröffentlichungen, sobald eine ausreichende Anzahl vorliegt, zu Handbuchbänden vereinigt, denen ein Register beigegeben wird. Der Verlag wird beim Erscheinen von Handbuchbänden den Buchhandel und die Interessenten darüber informieren, daß diese Handbuchbände eine Zusammenstellung bereits einzeln erschienener Monographien sind.

I. Introduction

The ECHO viruses (enteric cytopathogenic human orphan viruses) comprise a subgroup of the human enteroviruses: all are infectious for human beings. Although several may share common antigens, most are serologically unrelated. They have been grouped together with polio- and Coxsackie viruses because of similar physico-chemical properties, and because they are recoverable from the alimentary tract of human beings. Since 1951 when the first was recognized (ROBBINS et al., 1951), 32 more have been discovered. In recent years 2 members of the group have been placed in other categories: ECHO 10 is now reovirus type 1 (SABIN, 1959), and ECHO 28 is a rhinovirus, provisionally type 1 (TYRRELL and CHANOCK, 1963). During the last 15 years numerous studies have brought to light much information on the properties, ecology and natural history of the ECHO viruses.

II. Historical Résumé

Two conspicuous events fostered the rapid acquisition of knowledge of ECHO viruses. The first was a resurging interest in tissue culture methods permissive of viral growth *in vitro* (ENDERS et al., 1949); the second was the introduction of mass vaccination against poliomyelitis (FRANCIS et al., 1957). Both events enabled further recognition and delineation of the etiology of illnesses simulating nonparalytic poliomyelitis.

Beginning in 1950 cytopathogenic agents that were not polio- or Coxsackie viruses were encountered in the human alimentary tract (ROBBINS et al., 1951; KIBRICK and ENDERS, 1953; MELNICK, 1954; RAMOS-ALVAREZ and SABIN, 1954; HAMMON et al., 1955, 1957). A congeries of viruses thus became available during the next few years, thereby prompting a conference on orphan viruses (May, 1955, National Foundation for Infantile Paralysis, Inc.) and soon thereafter to the appointment of a Committee on the ECHO viruses of the National Foundation for Infantile Paralysis, whose main functions were definition of biological characteristics, and antigenic classes. Preliminary studies indicated the existence of multiple antigenic types; the first 13 serotypes were defined by exchange of prototype viruses and serum among the Committees' members. The orphan viruses were renamed the "enteric cytopathogenic human orphan (ECHO) group" and their properties defined about as follows: 1) they are cytopathogenic for monkey and human cells in culture; 2) they are not neutralized by poliovirus antisera; 3) they are not neutralized by antisera for Coxsackie viruses that are known to be cytopathogenic in tissue culture, and they fail to induce disease in infant mice; 4) they are not related to other groups of viruses recoverable from the alimentary tract (throat or intestines) by inoculation of primate tissue culture, such as herpes simplex, influenza, mumps, measles, varicella, adeno-, and (author's addition) the newly recognized myxoviruses (e.g. respiratory syncytial, parainfluenza, etc., among others); 5) they are neutralized by human gamma globulin and by individual human serums, thus indicating that they infect human beings (Committee on ECHO Viruses, 1955).

This Committee, acting as an unauthorized body, worked out some of the necessary approaches toward classification of this congeries of viruses, and was chiefly responsible for orderly progress in the field of enterovirus research. Once defined as "viruses in search of disease", since many were recovered from apparently healthy persons, most have found association with clinical disease. The original Committee sponsored by the National Foundation later acted (and continues to act) under the sponsorship of the National Institutes of Health (USA). Acting under various names (*Committee on ECHO Viruses; Committee on Enteroviruses;* and lastly *Committee on Human Picornaviruses*) the membership has changed periodically; nonetheless the fundamental guidelines remain much like those defined in 1955. As evidenced in the following pages, others have made fundamental contributions relating to basic physical properties, nature of viruses, serospecificity and association with clinical infection, all of which deservedly provide an interesting chapter in virology.

III. Classification and Nomenclature

The picornaviruses were so-named by an International Enterovirus Study Group (MELNICK et al., 1963) on the proviso that major groups of viruses have common biochemical and biophysical properties. Picornaviruses are small in size (15—30 mμ in diameter), are insensitive to ether, and contain ribonucleic acid cores. Cubic symmetry of the icosahedral type has been suggested as the structural form of some of these viruses, but few have been studied in detail; the number and arrangement of the capsomeres have not been established unequivocally. Enteroviruses are protected from thermal inactivation (50° C for 1 hour) by molar $MgCl_2$ and other salts of divalent cations (WALLIS and MELNICK, 1962).

Table 1. *The Picornaviruses*

I. Picornaviruses of human origin:

    A. Enteroviruses

        1. Polioviruses, types 1—3

        2. Coxsackie viruses A, types 1—24

        3. Coxsackie viruses B, types 1—6

        4. ECHO viruses, types 1—33

    B. Rhinoviruses

    C. Unclassified

II. Picornaviruses of lower animals:

    Includes the viruses of foot-and-mouth disease and Teschen disease, encephalomyelitis (Theiler's) and encephalomyelitis viruses of rodents, enteroviruses isolated from monkeys, cattle, swine, fowl, cats, etc., and rhinoviruses of equine bovine and other animal origin.

The derivation of the name picorna- is based as follows: pico, indicating very small viruses, and RNA, indicating that the genome contains ribonucleic acid; or alternatively, P, for polioviruses, the first known members of the group; i, for insensitivity to ether; c, for Coxsackie viruses, the second known member of the group; o for orphan viruses, the third subgroup, later named ECHO viruses; and r for rhinoviruses, the fourth subgroup.

At this point it is germane to review data recommended and data required (MELNICK et al., 1962; Committee on ECHO Viruses, 1955) for admission of new serotypes. Some of the recommendations relating to the enteroviruses have been lost to view in recent years, with the result that isolates reported as new serotypes are, on closer study, found to be either mixtures of viruses, or closely related if not identical members of recognized serotypes.

Data required for admission to the family of enteroviruses include the following: 1) *Evidence of human origin:* In addition to recovery of virus from the alimentary tract of one or more persons, type specific antibodies must be found in human sera (e.g. the donors, or in pooled gamma globulin). 2) *Resistance to ether:* Enteroviruses (as do all picornaviruses) retain full infectivity after treatment with 20% ethyl ether for 18 hours at 4° C; this is due to lack of essential lipids in virus structure. 3) *Size:* The particles shall range in size from 17—28 $m\mu$ as determined by electron microscopy, gradocol membrane filtration, or correspondingly reliable methods. 4) The single criterion currently useful in delineating entero- and rhinoviruses is the *acid-stability test;* enteroviruses suspended in fluids at pH values between 3 and 5 are stable, whereas rhinoviruses are not. However, results may not be always discriminatory. 5) *Serological distinction:* The new candidate shall be unrelated to previously recognized enteroviruses. The unknown virus ($\sim 100 \, \mathrm{TCID}_{50}$) shall be tested against reference antisera of all existing types. If antiserum pools, intersecting or otherwise are used, it is mandatory to repeat the test to confirm identity with a specific serum. Antisera against the unknown virus shall be prepared in animals and tested against prototypic virus strains. Mixtures containing two viruses have been troublesome; a requirement of new candidate viruses includes purification steps (triple plaque or terminal dilution passages) to assure homogeneity.

There are instances when additional data may be helpful. Such data include 1) character of cytopathogenic effect in tissue cultures, and/or pathological responses of animals (e.g. suckling mice and monkeys); 2) capacity to agglutinate erythrocytes; positive strains should be used in cross hemagglutination-inhibition tests with other enterovirus serotypes possessing this property; 3) if possible, a CF antigen for the candidate strain should be tested against type-specific sera for each previously recognized serotype; 4) the virus should contain ribonucleic acid, and 5) it should be stabilized to thermal inactivation in the presence of molar $MgCl_2$.

The Committee on Enteroviruses (USA) has been confronted with strains that do not fit comfortably into the subgroups noted in Table 1. Various strains within each subgroup produce in human beings identical neurological disease; still others produce respiratory, gastrointestinal and cutaneous lesions. Strains classified as ECHO viruses (e.g. type 9) cause myositis and paralysis in mice; some intratypic strains diverge widely in serological properties, or adapt with difficulty in tissue culture systems. Because of these fuzzy boundaries between members of subgroups the American Committee (MELNICK et al., 1962) suggested that recognized enteroviruses should be classified on an antigenic basis in a single numerical system. All newly recognized serotypes would be given a sequential enterovirus number. This proposal was not acceptable to many, including an International Study Group largely for two reasons: 1) identity dissociation based

Table 2. *The Prototypes of ECHO Viruses*

Type	Strain	Geographic origin	Illness in person yielding virus	Stocks Virus TCID$_{50}$ per ml log$_{10}$	Stocks Antisera Monkey sera SDE/ 0.1 ml
1	Farouk	Egypt	none	7.7	16,000
2	Cornelis	Connecticut	AM	5.8	12,600
3	Morrisey	Connecticut	AM	7.6	32,000
4	Pesascek	Connecticut	AM	5.0	90
5	Noyce	Maine	AM	8.7	22,000
6	D'Amori	Rhode Island	AM	8.3	40,000
6'	Cox	Ohio	none	4.8	2,800
6"	Burgess	Connecticut	AM	6.7	1,600
7	Wallace	Ohio	none	8.5	20,000
8	Bryson	Ohio	none	7.8	12,600
9	Hill	Ohio	none	7.3	32,000
11	Gregory	Ohio	none	7.3	6,400
12	Travis	Philippine Islands	none	9.0	22,000
13	Del Carmen	Philippine Islands	none	6.1	30,000
14	Tow	Rhode Island	AM	6.1	2,570
15	CH 96-51	West Virginia	none	5.2	1,260
16	Harrington	Massachusetts	AM	3.8	4,200
17	CHHE-29	Mexico City	none	5.4	2,000
18	Metcalf	Ohio	diarrhea	4.9	1,000
19	Burke	Ohio	diarrhea	7.4	16,000
20	JV-1	Washington, D.C.	fever	7.1	7,950
21	Farina	Massachusetts	AM	5.5	400
22	Harris	Ohio	diarrhea	6.7	20,000
23	Williamson	Ohio	diarrhea	—	32,000
24	DeCamp	Ohio	diarrhea	6.0	10,000
25	JV-4	Washington, D.C.	diarrhea	6.8	12,600
26	Coronel	Philippine Islands	none	6.3	8,000
27	Bacon	Philippine Islands	none	5.3	2,800
29	JV-10	Washington, D.C.	none	7.3	31,440
30	Bastianni	New York	AM	5.7	8,000
31	Caldwell	Kansas City, Kansas	AM	6.0	27,000
32	PR-10	Puerto Rico	AM	6.9	73,200
33	Toluca	Toluca, Mexico	none	6.8	260

—, irregular CPE.
TCID$_{50}$, 50% infective dose in cell cultures; SDE, serum dilution endpoint by neutralization test, expressed as reciprocal; AM, aseptic meningitis syndrome. The titration data entered in the last column are from the laboratories of the University of Kansas; some of the data have been reported (KAMITSUKA et al. Amer. J. Hyg. **74**, 7, 1961). The standardized monkey sera were prepared in these laboratories under the auspices of the National Foundation for Infantile Paralysis, Inc. (now the National Foundation, New York City) and the National Institutes of Health, Bethesda, Maryland, U.S.A. The investigators providing prototype strains are listed in the chapter on Enteroviruses, Diagnostic Procedures for Viral and Rickettsial Diseases, 3rd edition, Amer. publ. Hlth Ass. 1964 (MELNICK et al., 1964). Type 33, a recent serotype, has been characterized by ROSEN and KERN (Proc. Soc. exp. Biol. [N.Y.] **118**, 389, 1965).

on virological and clinical precedents, and 2) resistance to the "lumping" together of entero- and rhinoviruses. Like the American Committee the International Study Group were confronted with problems in classification, and assigned (on a temporary basis) new antigenic types in a subgroup, unclassified. At the present time, subclassification of picornaviruses requires the resolution of several conflicting points of view (ROSEN, 1965).

At the beginning when little was known concerning the viruses recovered from the human alimentary tract by cell culture techniques, there was reason to call them "orphans". Their small size (in contrast to adenoviruses, which may also be found in feces) lack of pathogenicity for suckling mice, and serological distinction from polio- and Coxsackie viruses provided several distinctions, and in the absence of other criteria many were placed in the ECHO category where they remain pending resolution of problems noted above. At this time there are 31 serotypes. A listing of the prototype strains, a part of their histories, and several properties of each appear in Table 2.

IV. Virus Replication

A. Susceptibility of Cultured Cells

1. Cytopathogenic Effect

Most ECHO viruses multiply, producing typically destructive cytopathogenic effect (CPE) in primary cultures of primate kidney cells. Rhesus (*Macaca mulatta*) and cynomolgus *(M. cynomolgus)* kidney cells are almost uniformly susceptible (except type 21), as are similar cells of African green *(Cercopithecus aethiops sabaeus)* and tantalus *(C. aethiops tantalus)* monkeys, and the baboon *(Papio doguero)* (HSIUNG and MELNICK, 1957a, b; HSIUNG, 1962; KALTER et al., 1962). Kidney cells of the red grass monkey *(Erythrocebus patas)* are susceptible to lysis by types 7, 8, 12, 19, 22, 23, 24, and 25, and have been used to delineate biological groupings. The LLC-MK$_2$ continuous line of monkey kidney cells (HULL et al., 1962) is less useful for primary isolation of ECHO viruses (HAMBLING and DAVIS, 1965).

ECHO viruses are also cytopathogenic for a variety of human cells cultured *in vitro*, these include primary cultures of human amnion, kidney and thyroid (LAHELLE, 1957; LEHMANN-GRUBE, 1961; LEE et al., 1965; DUNCAN, 1960), and serially cultured human diploid (embryonic lung) (HAYFLICK and MOORHEAD, 1961) and aorta cell strains (BEHBEHANI et al., 1965). Continuous lines of cells (e.g. HeLa, KB, Maben, HEp-2, Detroit 196 Fb-L) are usually less sensitive than primary cells, however, there are exceptions (ARCHETTI et al., 1957; PAL et al., 1963). Continuous lines of cells having the morphological appearance of fibroblasts are more susceptible to these viruses than are epithelial-like cells (STULBERG et al., 1958).

The gross cytopathic effects in primate cells engendered by enteroviruses include a sequence of cellular changes characterized by increased refractivity, retraction of cell margins, nuclear distortion, cytoplasmic granularity followed by contortion and lysis of cells. Sequential changes observable in unstained cultures by ordinary light microscopy are similar for almost all enteroviruses, excepting a prolongation of the lag-phase for ECHO and Coxsackie virus subgroups.

Cytological changes associated with types 22 and 23 differ from those thus far found for other enteroviruses. The earliest changes resemble those encountered

Table 3. Origin of Cells and Susceptibility to CPE by ECHO Viruses

Animals			Kind of cell cultures	Cellular response			Remarks
Order	Genus	Species		Primary CPE	CPE on adaptation	No primary CPE	
Primates	Man	Homo sapiens	Kidney — P	+++	—	—	excellent response
			Amnion — P	± to +++	—	—	variable response
			Thyroid — P	+++	—	—	excellent response
			HeLa — C	± to ++++	+++	+	variable response[1]
			Detroit 196	+ to ++++	+++	?	for types 1 to 16
			WI-38	+ to +++	—	—	good, including type 21
			HEp-2	0	?+	+	for types 1—3 and 5—24
	Monkey	M. mulatta	Kidney — P	+++	—	—	excellent response, except type 21
		M. cynomolgus	Kidney — P	+++	—	—	excellent response, except type 21
		C. aethiops sabeus	Kidney — P	++	—	—	excellent response, except type 21
		E. patas	Kidney — P	types 7, 12, 19 and 22—25	?	+	variable, even in responsive sero-types
	Baboon	P. doguera	Kidney — P	+ to +++	types 1, 3, 13, 23, 24 and 26	types 2, 14 and 21	variable response
Lower verte-brates	Hamster	C. auratus	Kidney — P	0	± types 4, 9		for types 1—19
	Swine	—	Kidney — P	0	+ type 4		for types 1—9, 11, and 14—19
					± type 9		

[1] Several lines of HeLa cells are known to vary in susceptibility to enteroviruses. We have obtained CPE with E 9 on calf kidney cells, after several blind passages.

P, primary cell cultures; C, continuous cell lines; primary CPE refers to the effect obtained on first passage of virus in these cells; usually not necessary to passage for adaptation, but see text for comments regarding types 22 and 23; ? data needed for clarification of issue.

with other serotypes; they are set apart by nuclear alterations appearing later in infection (WIGAND and SABIN, 1961; SHAVER et al., 1961; WENNER, 1962a). The nucleolus fades and disappears. Chromatin granules aggregate at the periphery of the nucleus; the intranuclear structures leach away (between 8 and 20 hours) leaving a refractile, rounded cell and an "empty-appearing" nucleus. Infected cells stained with acridine orange show alterations of normal green fluorescence (DNA) of nuclei and orange-red fluorescence of nucleoli. Green fluorescence only is found in chromatin granules and thickened nuclear membranes. Empty nuclei contain a faint gray-green reticular network.

Cultured cells ordinarily fully sensitive to the CPE of most ECHO viruses may sometimes be refractory for primary isolations. This refractory state, which may persist for several serial passages, has been encountered among some type 22 and 23 strains (WIGAND and SABIN, 1961) among others. Sometimes CPE is more easily demonstrated in human amnion than in monkey kidney cells. The precise reasons for the relative refractory state have not been defined, but may relate to the receptor (attachment) sites, defects in virus assembly, serum inhibitors, or other alterations (acidity) of cellular milieu (BARRON and KARZON, 1957).

2. Cell Pathology

When cells obtained at various stages of infections are carefully fixed and appropriately stained, it is possible to delineate a series of morphological events (BERNKOPF and ROSIN, 1957; BUCKLEY, 1956, 1957; SHAVER et al., 1958; BARSKI, 1962; GODMAN et al., 1964a). With ECHO 9, earliest discernible changes occur at the cytoplasmic rim of the nucleus as a zone of increased basophilia. Nuclear alterations include the early development of eosinophilic granules ($\sim$4 hours) which increase for a short interval ($\sim$8 hours) and then decline. At mid-stage the nucleus is distorted, ridged (chromatin filaments) and plicated. Soon after the appearance of perinuclear basophilia, a homogeneous pale mass accumulates in a juxtanuclear position, displacing and compressing basophilic components now chiefly localized in the mantle zone of the cytoplasm. Other coincidental developments include retraction and rounding of cells, formation of cytoplasmic vacuoles, nodular cytoplasmic protrusions, shedding of vacuoles and ecdysis of the basophilic mantle. Among these alterations the basophilic aggregates have been correlated with viral antigen using fluorescence-labeled antibody (BUCKLEY, 1957; GODMAN et al., 1964a).

The application of cytochemical methods, autoradiography, and phase contrast, fluorescence (fluorochromes and labeled antibody) and electron microscopy (SHAVER et al., 1958; RIFKIND et al., 1961; JAMESON et al., 1963; GODMAN et al., 1964b) has provided further insight of alterations within the cell. By midphase ($\sim$12 to 24 hours) cells exhibiting the peripheral basophilic rim begin coalescence of the juxtanuclear mass. The juxtanuclear mass appears to consist of collections of smooth walled vesicles, some of high lipid content, some empty-appearing and all of low fluorescence with labeled antibody. Basophilic components are chiefly ribosomes, displaced by the juxtanuclear mass, they gather into large and small aggregates, or are arrayed in short linear series in various strata of the cytoplasm. Immunofluorescent studies of similar changes with poliovirus (BUCKLEY, 1957) suggest an association of viral antigen with the basophilic components, presumably the ribosomes. Fine granular deposits of electron dense material, and fine filaments of size similar to the fibrils separating viral particles appear in the cytoplasm. Shortly after the emergence of the juxtanuclear mass (the time varies due to asynchronous cell-infection cycles) and coincidental with aggregation of ribosomes, aggregates of viral particles (22 to 24 mμ) appear at the edge of the juxtanuclear mass, and elsewhere in the cytoplasm. Mitochondria, as noted by others (SHAVER et al., 1958) are also concentrated in the region of the juxtanuclear mass. RIFKIND et al. (1961) described dense granular particles (12—18 mμ) regularly arrayed on the inner cristae of these organelles.

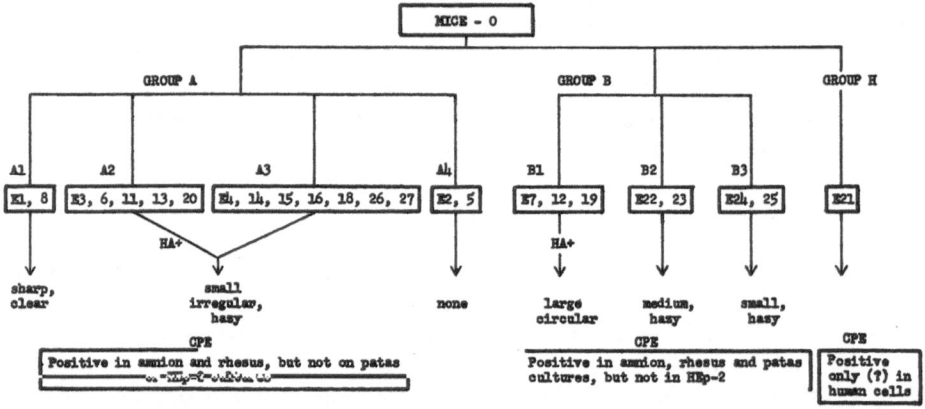

Fig. 1. Schema for grouping ECHO viruses based on plaque patterns and CPE in tissue cultures. Subgroups A and B are based on plaque patterns and hemagglutination property. Hemagglutinating properties have been observed for serotypes in subgroups A 2 and B1. Reliance on grouping is based on the pattern, and has been of value for preliminary identification. Strain variations within serotypes have been observed. ECHO 19 requires large inocula. Some of these findings are not in agreement with those published by MAISEL and MOSCOVICI (1961). Modified from Fig. 4 of G.D. HSIUNG, Ann. N.Y. Acad. Sci. 101, 419 (1962).

B. Plaque Formation

1. Morphology

When all conditions have been satisfied (dose, type of cell, agar overlay, etc.) most ECHO viruses implanted on monolayers of monkey kidney cells produce visible plaques (areas of cell necrosis or virus colonies). Plaque morphology varies not only between serotypes, but also among strains of the same type (MAISEL and MOSCOVICI, 1961). Despite these variations, plaque morphology has been used along with several other criteria for differentiation of enteroviruses. Excepting type 21, all ECHO viruses produce plaques on kidney cells of rhesus monkeys. For some ECHO viruses the plaques are small, irregular and hazy and may not be readily separable into serological classes. These viruses multiply slowly, attaining plaque diameters of 0.5 cm by the 10th day. For others plaques are large, circular and clear resembling those encountered with wild-type polioviruses. Such viruses grow rapidly, reach 1 cm or more in diameter a week after seeding.

Plaque development is enhanced by the presence of $MgCl_2$ (WALLIS et al., 1962). As was noted above kidney cells from patas monkeys are not susceptible to CPE by all ECHO viruses. Patas-positive strains are also characterized by variation in plaque morphology, and occasionally (ECHO 19) plaques form only when large inocula are used. HSIUNG has used plaque morphology and host-cell infectivity spectra as a basis for grouping enteroviruses (HSIUNG and MELNICK, 1957 a, b; HSIUNG, 1962). The schema used to delineate biological groupings of ECHO viruses based on mouse pathogenicity, plaque morphology, host-cell infectivity spectra, and hemagglutination is outlined in Fig. 1.

The plaque method is more sensitive than the conventional CPE method for counting virus particles, delineating low levels of antibody (e.g. ECHO 4), recovery of "pure" clones, and as an assay method of infectivity of viral RNA. A microplaque method has been used advantageously by SOMMERVILLE (1959).

2. Inhibitors

The presence of sulfated polysaccharides in commercially available agar used in the preparation of overlay media is known to inhibit the development of enterovirus plaques (TAKEMOTO and LIEBHABER, 1961; BARRON and KARZON, 1962). This inhibitory effect can be nullified by the incorporation of polycations diethyl-aminoethyl (DEAE) dextran or protamine. Plaque diameters of types 5, 8, 11 and 26 are considerably increased by addition of DEAE-dextran to the agar overlay, while the completion of CPE by these types is slowed by dextran sulfate and agar extract (ROUHANDEH et al., 1965). The mechanism underlying this inhibition has not yet been elucidated. However, it has been shown that the intracellular growth of poliovirus strain LSc 2 ab was not inhibited by sulfated polysaccharides but its adsorption to susceptible cells was prevented, thereby suggesting that an ionic interaction binds or restricts the virus (LIEBHABER and TAKEMOTO, 1963; BENGTSSON, 1965).

Inhibition of CPE (types 7, 9, and 19) and plaque formation (types 7 and 19) have been observed in primary rhesus monkey kidney cells overlaid with fluids and cellular extracts of several continuous cell lines, e.g., HeLa, Detroit-6, KB, HEp-2, FL. This inhibition was ascribed to a factor called "inhibitor of viral activity" and could be assayed quantitatively by its inhibitory effect on type 7 plaques. No such inhibitor could be detected in primary monkey kidney, human fibroblastic and certain other malignant or primary non-primate cell cultures (TSILINSKY, 1963a). The inhibitory effect was associated with filtrable particles which sedimented at 22,000 g in 2 hours. Trypsin, heating at 68° C and UV irradiation destroyed the activity. The inhibitors originated in the cytoplasm (not in the nucleus), gradually increased with incubation and accumulated in the overlay fluid through release from the cells (TSILINSKY, 1963b). Cell cultures prepared from different monkeys had different sensitivity levels to the inhibitors. The interaction between cells and inhibitors resulted in the adsorption of inhibitors and their disappearance since they could not subsequently be recovered from either the cells or the fluids. Cell cultures coming in contact with inhibitors (80 minutes at 37° C) prior to virus infection also exhibited antiviral activity (TSILINSKY, 1963c). Although the continuous cell lines producing the inhibitors were contaminated with PPLO, this contamination was apparently not responsible for the inhibitory effects of these cultures (TSI-LINSKY and LEVASHEV, 1963). It was also observed that treatment of primary monkey kidney cells with these inhibitors (45 minutes at 37° C) caused a significant delay in the nonspecific degeneration (TSILINSKY, 1963d).

C. Mechanisms of Cellular Infection

ECHO viruses interact *in vitro* with cultured cells, reproduce and destroy the host. The steps in this dynamic process, involving attachment, penetrance, reception, reproduction, assembly and release of new viral particles have been explored during the past decade mainly for the polioviruses. Similar phases in the development of the virion presumably apply to the ECHO viruses; at best they seem to for those that have been studied. The basic properties of the virion are best understood on a bedrock of knowledge concerning morphological and biochemical events during the replicative cycle. At this point then we shall be concerned largely but not exclusively with the total cellucidal impact, fully recognizing that various means of dampening cytopathogenicity are matters also of considerable interest.

1. Attachment and Penetration

Mechanisms of attachment and penetration of ECHO viruses have not been studied as carefully as those of polioviruses. Cell receptors provide sites of virus attachment. Surface attachment is independent of temperature and reversible, whereas "penetrance" (and eclipse) is temperature-dependent and irreversible (HOLLAND, 1962). During this latter stage it appears that viral RNA is released for entry into the cells' nucleic acid pool where the message is decoded.

Receptors located on intact cell membranes are essential for irreversible viral attachment. All fully sensitive primate cells have them. Cells in organized tissues of intact animals (e.g. monkey kidney) normally resistant to infection acquire susceptibility to enteroviruses *in vitro*. Receptor activity has not been found among enterovirus-insensitive cells derived from dog, cat, swine, calf, guinea pig, mouse, chick or rabbit (McLAREN et al., 1959), although such cells may be competent to support virus replication if intact virus or its infective RNA reaches the interior of the cell (HOLLAND et al., 1959). However, the in-susceptibility of cells derived from enterovirus-insensitive mammals is not absolute; cellulicidal effects have been obtained with Group B Coxsackie viruses on kidney cells of swine, lamb, and hamster (LENAHAN and WENNER, 1960). Among ECHO viruses types 1, 4, and 9, that were tested only type 4 produced CPE in swine cells. Others (GUERIN and GUERIN, 1957; BARRON and KARZON, 1959; CRANDELL et al., 1961) either failed to obtain CPE, or noted only minimal activity. The unique susceptibilities of these cells *extra situ* may stem in the overgrowth of undifferentiated cell types which acquire surface receptors thereby providing the means of initiating successful intracellular infection (KUNIN, 1962). DARNELL and SAWYER (1960) suggested that the basis for variation in sus-ceptibility of resistant cells (HeLa) was related, not to reversible eclipse during attachment, but to a relative inefficiency of release of viral RNA from the protein coat after penetration of the virion. Evidence of virus breakdown at the cell surface, with alteration of surface protein of the virus, suggested as a prelude to release of viral RNA (JOKLIK and DARNELL, 1961), may be an important factor in abortive virus-cell interactions.

PHILIPSON and LIND (1964) demonstrated irreversible union of ECHO 7 virus to soluble receptors of erythrocyte membranes, which is temperature dependent, has sharp pH optimum, and appears to be a first order reaction. This interaction, assumed to be enzymatic is followed by release of infectious RNA, which is an event differing from the interaction of poliovirus with surface receptors (plasma membranes) wherein viral RNA is not released from the capsid (HOLLAND and HOYER, 1962).

Sulfhydryl groups are involved in the adsorption of certain enteroviruses to monkey kidney cells. During adsorption of some enteroviruses onto cultures of monkey kidney cells, sulfhydryl groups may react with a disulfide group on the susceptible cell in the form of sulfhydryl-disulfide interchange. The sulfhydryl reagent, p-chloromercuribenzoate (PCMB) inactivates both hemagglutinin and infectivity by preventing viral adsorption. These effects of PCMB are reversed by glutathione — a thiol compound. The rate of inactivation of viral infectivity of PCMB was markedly affected by the purity of virus, the buffer used and the pH. Reactivation of infectivity by the thiol compound was also affected by certain conditions; reactivation was not consistently reversed by glutathione in the presence of high concentrations of PCMB, prolonged treatment at 37° C or phosphate buffer (in lieu of tris-buffered saline) (CHOPPIN and PHILIPSON, 1961). A number of other viruses are unaffected by sulfhydryl reagents indicating a distinct but as yet ill-defined mode of attachment for sensitive viruses.

Cell cultures exposed to anticellular serum may be protected with respect to CPE for certain ECHO viruses (HABEL et al., 1958; QUERSIN-THIRY, 1958). Antisera prepared in rabbits against either cultured or uncultured human amnion cells are cytotoxic for human amnion cells, inhibit plaque formation by certain ECHO viruses (in human amnion monolayers), agglutinate human erythrocytes, and fix complement (antibody for amnion cells). The inhibitory effect of these antisera on plaque formation was due to their action on cells, presumably the receptors and not by neutralization of the virus. Antiserum produced against cultured cells reduced the plaque count 85% for serotypes 1, 7, and 9, while antisera produced against uncultured cells gave an average reduction of 33%. When cultured cell antiserum was absorbed with human O erythrocytes, or with uncultured amnion cells, the inhibitory effect dropped from 85 to 55%. Absorption of serum with cultured amnion cells completely removed the inhibitory effect. The uncultured cell antiserum was rendered completely devoid of any inhibitory effect by adsorption with human red cells or cultured or uncultured amnion cells. It was concluded that the cultured cell antiserum possessed antibodies against two different antigens, namely, one present only in cultured cells and the other in human erythrocytes and both cultured and uncultured cells. Most of the inhibitory effect of cultured cell antiserum was thus due to antibodies against the antigen present only in cultured cells (the antigen being acquired during culture). Furthermore, differences in the inhibitory effect of anticellular sera on various members of the enterovirus group (polio- and Coxsackie viruses B were generally not inhibited) gave evidence that immunologically distinct cell receptors may be involved in the adsorption of enteroviruses to susceptible cells (TIMBURY, 1962, 1963).

In contrast with the information accumulated on the factors facilitating or blocking virus adsorption, the mechanisms used by enteroviruses to penetrate the cell wall are largely unknown. Evidence of enzymatic activity between virus and cell has been suggested, but no correlation between enzymes and penetrance has been established. Virus may enter cells by pinocytosis or viropexis.

2. Reproduction

The intracellular replication of viral protein and RNA are independent events; subunits are formed at different rates and probably at different intracellular sites. These subunits assemble to form the complete virion (or under specified circumstances, incomplete virus). Intracellular sites of assembly are in the cytoplasm, presumably in close association with ribosomal aggregates. Preformed components of the cell's nucleotide pool are used for synthesizing viral RNA (SALZMAN and SEBRING, 1961) as are cell proteins (amino-acids) for synthesizing the protein coat. Interruption of DNA synthesis has no effect on reproduction of RNA viruses; however, it is not known whether viral RNA must first replicate (or decode without replication) in the nucleus and then transfer to the cytoplasm where it serves as template. Intracellular replication occurs swiftly; poliovirus RNA and protein synthesis appear to take place simultaneously, for RNA peak concentrations precede viral maturation by about an hour.

The reproduction of the majority of ECHO viruses is specifically inhibited by 2-(α-hydroxybenzyl)-benzimidazole (HBB) and guanidine (EGGERS and TAMM, 1961; TAMM and EGGERS, 1962, 1963; RIGHTSEL et al., 1961). These two compounds, at concentrations which markedly inhibit virus reproduction have no significant effects on the biosynthetic and energy-yielding activities of cell cultures. However, in infected cultures, each selectively inhibits the synthesis of virus-induced RNA polymerase (the enzyme system necessary for the synthesis of viral RNA), and of viral capsid protein subunits. Furthermore, each markedly reduces viral CPE in infected cultures. The adsorption and release of virus, however, are not affected and no inactivating effect on virus particles or infective viral RNA is observed.

Except types 22 and 23, all other ECHO viruses are susceptible to HBB and guanidine HCl; both types 22 and 23 are insusceptible to either compound (TAMM and EGGERS, 1962). Both compounds together produce a synergistic effect — the combination being more inhibitory than doubling the concentration of each alone (EGGERS and TAMM, 1963a). Only partial cross resistance has been observed between the two compounds (TAMM and EGGERS, 1962). With large inocula of a susceptible ECHO virus and low concentrations of inhibitor (especially guanidine), breakthrough occurs, with the emergence of stable resistant mutants (EGGERS and TAMM, 1961). It has been suggested that the emergence of resistant mutants depends on HBB serving as both a selective agent and a facilitator or an inducer of resistant particles. In addition to resistant mutants, drug-dependent particles are also encountered (EGGERS and TAMM, 1963b). As in resistance, dependence also relates to the genetic profile of the virion; in the absence of the drug the synthesis of virus-induced RNA polymerase as well as viral RNA is inhibited for drug-dependent progeny (EGGERS et al., 1963; BALTIMORE et al., 1963). Back mutation to either drug resistance, or to drug dependence may occur. One out of every 1000—5000 particles, produced in HBB-dependent ECHO virus type 13 infected cultures, is drug-independent (EGGERS and TAMM, 1963 b).

The events in the selective inhibitory effect of these compounds for the reproduction of picornaviruses are still obscure. The two compounds differ from one another in molecular size, aromaticity, basicity, number of nitrogen atoms and steric points. They have different spectra of virus-inhibiting actions on various members of the picornavirus group. Minor modification in their structure can remove their inhibitory action. One common feature between the two compounds is the $>N-\acute{C}=N-$ sequence and this has been suggested to be a possible essential feature for the specific inhibitory effect of these compounds (TAMM and EGGERS, 1963). But it is unknown whether the inhibitory effect takes place at a common locus in the cell.

3. Assembly and Release

The visible packaging of enteroviruses in crystalline arrays, and their unordered (which may be only apparent) distribution in the cytoplasm suggest maturation in association with ergoplasmic membranes. We noted earlier the independency of viral protein and RNA synthesis; data on assembly of the enteroviruses suggest also that the protein of the capsomeres and viral RNA may be synthesized in close proximity of the other.

While the assembly of virions assumes interdependence of nucleic acid and protein synthesis, HALPEREN et al. (1964a) demonstrated with ECHO 12 that virus protein synthesis and capsid assembly are independent of nucleic acid synthesis. By sequential treatment of infected cells with 2-(α-hydroxybenzyl)-benzimidazole (HBB) (an inhibitor of viral RNA polymerase and RNA synthesis) and DL-p-fluorophenylalanine (FPA) (at the right concentration FPA inhibits production of infectious virus, while synthesis of infectious viral RNA continues at a reduced rate) they showed an arrest in synthesis of the virion with FPA, and continued production of capsid protein with HBB. Thus, it would appear that viral RNA produced in the presence of FPA before addition of HBB served as messenger RNA in the limited synthesis of empty capsid protein.

The cytochemical transformations obtained during infection with ECHO 9 virus were interpreted as follows by GODMAN et al. (1964b). Shortly after infection, there was prompt cessation of DNA synthesis, without net change, and loss of nonhistone protein by distorted nuclei. There was flocculation of intranuclear chromatin and cessation of incorporation of isotopic precursors of RNA in the nucleus. During the first half of the infection cycle, no change occurred in the net amount of RNA per cell. Infection prevented uptake of nucleocapside precursors in the formation of all RNAs (ribosomal RNA, messenger RNA) that are normally synthesized in the nucleus. In contrast, incorporation of the precursors into RNA in the cytoplasm, in or upon cellular ribosomes, was initiated. The newly synthesized RNA was equated with the infectious RNA. The viral protein, apparently synthesized in the ribosomal aggregates as determined by the fluorescent antibody technique, was invariably associated with the basophilic ribonucleoprotein aggregations. The postulate was that *the infectious RNA* acts as an extrinsic messenger RNA possessing the necessary information for the synthesis of viral protein subunits as well as being able to catalyze its own replication by the use of cellular ribosomes. The synthesis of viral protein (and probably viral RNA) preceded the appearance of viral particles; apparently until production of these subcomponents was far in excess of that utilized for the formation of all viral progeny. TOLBERT et al. (1966) found similar relationships for ECHO 19. Viral assembly (packing together of viral RNA and viral protein capsid) took place in finely granular material of undetermined composition at sites spatially removed from sites involved in the synthesis of the two moieties. In the center of infected cells, a chromophobic mass consisting of phospholipid-rich smooth-walled membranes and vesicles was observed. The masses were considered to be probably newly synthesized phospholipoprotein. The new phospholipid synthesis as well as the observed increased lipid phosphorylation were thought to be probably associated with the shedding phenomenon at the cell surface (similar to cell membrane transport). The vesicles composed the juxtanuclear mass and some of them had concentric double or multiple lamellas. Many vesicles contained large dense granules. While mitochondrial succinic dehydrogenase and adenosinetriphosphatase activities continued high, the nucleosidediphosphatase activity associated with the internal membrane vanished in infected cells. The relationship of the mitochondrial particles to intracellular virus multiplication is unknown.

By definition (LWOFF, 1957), as true viruses, ECHO viruses contain only RNA, multiply from their RNA and do not possess energy-generating enzymes. If the replicative steps are analogous to other RNA viruses (i.e. poliovirus, mengovirus) the single-stranded RNA of ECHO viruses must possess the necessary information for the biosynthesis of at least three macromolecular components involved in the production of new virions. These components are viral RNA, viral protein subunits of the capsid and specific enzymes catalyzing the biochemical reactions leading to the production of the viral progeny. During the viral biosynthetic process, the first new sets of components to appear (about two hours after cellular infection) are certain proteins which are unrelated to viral capsid proteins but most probably contain the specific viral RNA catalyzing enzyme polymerase. Since the only known mechanism by which nucleic acids can replicate is by base-pair copying, it is postulated that intercellularly, during the replicating stage the single-stranded RNA of picornaviruses takes the form of a double-stranded RNA, and with the catalyzation of viral RNA polymerase, new viral RNA is synthesized. Such double-stranded viral RNA has been detected in cell cultures infected with polio- and EMC viruses (MONTAGNIER and SANDERS, 1963; BALTIMORE et al., 1964; PONS, 1964). The third component, namely viral capsid protein, is assembled in a series of steps in which viral RNA itself serves as the messenger RNA (the messenger RNA in DNA viruses is produced by virus-specific messenger RNA through the catalyzation of DNA polymerases) and acts as template for the synthesis of the protein subunits. The consecutive sequence of each of three of the four nucleotide bases (adenine, guanidine, cytosine and uracil) of the messenger RNA, determines the identity of a single amino acid in the corresponding site of the long polypeptide chain of the protein subunit. The complete virions develop presumably through a process of self-assembly (the directions for which are built into the structures of the components) uniting together viral protein subunits and specific nucleic acid molecules (GREEN, 1965; TAMM and EGGERS, 1965).

V. Properties

A. Physical Structure

1. Purified Virus Preparations

An outstanding characteristic of most animal viruses is their stability and capacity to survive often rigorous procedures used for partition of macromolecules. Several methods are based on variations in physical properties (e.g. size, density and molecular weight), whereas others are based on differences in physicochemical properties (surface configuration, etc.). By using one or more of these methods it is possible to separate the viral particle from much of the extraneous non-viral components of the milieu. Ultracentrifugation (with or without density gradient columns) and zone electrophoresis have been applied to enteroviruses, either to obtain samples containing the virion, or subcomponents thereof. POLSON and DEEKS (1962), using zone electrophoresis found that the majority of polio- and Coxsackie viruses migrated slowly, whereas several ECHO viruses migrated more rapidly in the electric field. HOYER et al. (1958) obtained a marked purification of P^{32}-labeled ECHO virus type 13 using ECTEOLA-SF cellulose ion exchanger. The order in which polio- and ECHO 9 viruses were eluted from the ECTEOLA column corresponded with their mobilities in the electric field (POLSON and DEEKS, 1962). As might be expected, the elution of viruses, including strains of the same type, may have differing patterns. The surface configuration of the prototypic ECHO virus type 4 (Pesascek) appears to differ from that of the homotypic Dutoit, in that the former exchanged for phosphate on anion resin columns whereas the latter did not (WALLIS et al., 1965). Other complexes, such as activated attapulgate, a hydrated magnesium-aluminium silicate, have been used for adsorbing ECHO viruses (BARTELL et al., 1960).

ECHO virus types 7 and 19 have been purified and concentrated ($\geq 1000 \times$) by two-phase system of dextran sulfate-polyethylene glycol or polyvinyl alcohol; a particular advantage is that concentration is obtained without the potential damaging effects of ultracentrifugation (PHILIPSON et al., 1960). In later studies of ECHO 7 virus labeled with P^{32}, PHILIPSON and LIND (1964) passed the virus material through a column of Sephadex G-100 to remove further impurities prior to separation by high speed centrifugation after layering on CsCl. The sharp separation, based on assay of each fraction for radioactivity, infectivity and hemagglutinin, is illustrated in Fig. 2. The overall recovery of virus infectivity was 74% of the original, and the purification factor was 650. KITANO et al. (1961) pointing out that a complete separation of virus from serum protein may not be achieved used an organic solvent (2-ethoxyethanol and 2-butoxyethanol) for separation of ECHO 7 virus. Appropriate mixtures of infected tissue culture fluid, phosphate solution (~ 2.5 M K_2HPO_4, pH 7.5) and organic solvent were centrifuged, yielding a gel-like interface containing infective virus concentrated 20- to 100-fold per milligram protein.

2. Morphology

Early work involving irradiation with electrons, alpha particles and deuterons as means of measuring the size of irradiation-sensitive units of ECHO virus types 1 and 7 indicated diameters ranging between 24 and 32 mμ; ultrafiltration procedures measuring the whole particle size gave values within the same range (BENYESH et al., 1958). However, in gradacol-membrane filtration tests with several ECHO viruses, the size was 18 mμ or less (SABIN, 1959).

Particle sizes determined by electron microscopy fall within the same range. Ultrathin sections of a highly purified ECHO virus type 7 preparation contained viral particles in crystalline array with average dimensions of 17×22 mμ (HANZON

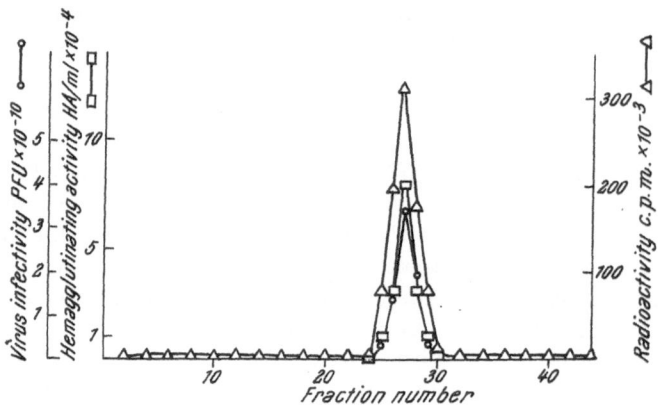

Fig. 2. Preparation of purified ECHO virus type 7 labeled with P³². Density gradient centrifugation in CsCl. Peak activities, assayed for radioactivity, infectivity and hemagglutinin coincide in the density gradient. The fraction containing the maximum activity had a buoyant density of 1.36 g./ml. After L. PHILIPSON and M. LIND, Virology **23**, 322—332 (1964).

and PHILIPSON, 1960). Similar findings relate to type 4 (DUFFEY et al., 1962), type 9 (RIFKIND et al., 1961), type 30 (DUNCAN and TIMBURY, 1961) and an unclassified "ECHO virus" (STUART et al., 1960).

The morphological structure of ECHO viruses during assembly in infected cells has been examined at different levels of development. The differences encountered between serotypes relate to stages of maturation, preparation methods (fixation, embedding, staining and shadowing) and the elucidation of fine structure by electron micrography.

The earliest changes in monkey kidney cells infected with type 4 (DUFFEY et al., 1962) correspond with those noted earlier for ECHO virus type 9. Aggregates of virus particles (~ 20 mμ) appear in the cytoplasm, some as a crystalline lattice, others in linear array, and still others distributed randomly in the cytoplasm. Some particles were encased by a limiting membrane with or without a dense nucleoid (6 mμ); other particles without such membranes exhibited great variation in size (≤ 20 mμ), shape and electron density. Several additional findings were obtained with type 9 (RIFKIND et al., 1961) where also non-crystalline parallel rows of particles were seen in the cytoplasm, the majority of the particles were dense, with a linear center-to-center distance of about 25 mμ. These linear bead-like arrays were separated by linear filaments (2—5 mμ in diameter and several microns in length). Further studies indicated the particulate structure to consist of a dense central structure (13—15 mμ in diameter) surrounded by a delicate outer membrane. Direct measurement of individual particles indicated a size of 22 mμ. Incomplete particles apparently lacking the central core were seen only in the cytoplasm. Extracellular particles of similar size, and containing dense central cores were seen outside the cells. In another study (NUÑEZ-MONTIEL et al., 1961) 3 kinds of particles were found in the cytoplasm of monkey kidney cells infected with ECHO viruses. The particles most clearly depicted were homogeneous in appearance, uniform in size and arrayed as crystals. Such particles were observed in cells infected with types 6 and 19, but not in cells infected with type 9. The particles had an osmiophilic central dense mass, and were surrounded by an electron lucid zone with an average size of 14.4 mμ for type 6, and 14.5 for type 19. The crystals were clustered into hexagonal packages, forming angles of 75° and 105° (never 90°). The particles were arranged in rows separated by a constant distance (about 1.5—2.5 times the distance between particles) which differed from one crystal to another. The distance between the individual particles was also constant in each crystal but differed from one crystal to another and ranged from 20—30 mμ. Two other kinds of particles observed in the infected cells were: a) smaller units, arranged in clusters (never in crystals) and measuring about 10 mμ, which were considered to be nucleoprotein granules; b) larger units, quite dense with clear borders and measuring from 20—50 mμ. The latter were rarely seen, usually occurred singly and were considered unrelated to virus (possibly a product of cellular disintegration). A similar electron microscopic study (JAMISON et al., 1963) of monkey kidney cells infected with two strains (Pesascek and Dutoit) of ECHO virus type 4 gave essentially the same results. However, while Dutoit-infected cells showed particles in close-packed crystals, the particles of Pesascek-infected cells were in disorganized clusters. Both particles were of the same size (17—19 mμ as determined by center-to-center measurement). More recently the viral symmetry of ECHO virus types 4, 11, and 24 was studied (MAYOR, 1964). These viruses were purified by density gradient centrifugation in CsCl and concentrated by pelleting at 40,000 r.p.m. The viral preparations were mixed with equal volumes of 1% phosphotungstic acid (at pH 7.0) and placed on carbon-coated grids for electron microscopy. In order to resolve the fine morphology of the viral capsid (protein coat), certain individual particles which appeared in sharp contrast against a background of phosphotungstic acid were selected for the preparation of enlarged photographic reversals. In such preparations, particle diameters measured from 20—24 mμ. Most viral particles exhibited an architecture of 2 five-fold axes of cubic symmetry formed on the opposite vertexes of a conspicuous central rhombus. The capsids, thus appeared to consist of 32 capsomeres arranged in the form of a rhombic triacontahedron rather than a regular icosahedron.

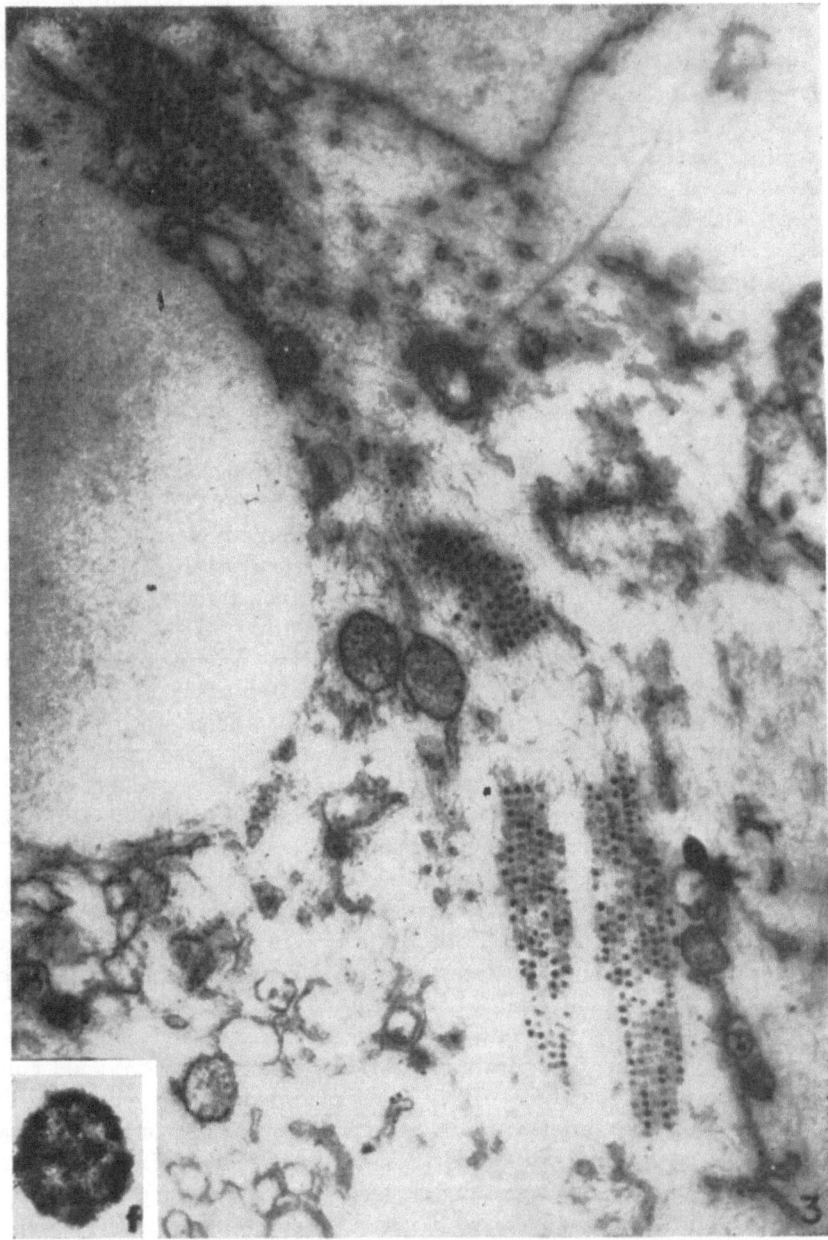

Fig. 3. Linear arrays of ECHO virus type 9 in an infected cell. Electron micrograph, ×58,300. After
R. A. RIFKIND et al., J. exp. Med. 114, 1 −12 (1961). The virus particle in the lower left corner is ECHO
virus 24. Electron micrograph, printed in reverse contrast ×750,000. After H. D. MAYOR, Virology 22,
156 −160 (1964).

All studies place the ECHO viruses among the smallest of the known human viruses; while the exact number and arrangement of their protein subunits have not been definitely established for many, it appears that the structural units (capsomeres) of ECHO virus virions are assembled in identical symmetry, with definite configuration.

B. Chemical Structure

The current image of a viral particle is of a species of nucleic acid wrapped in its protein coat. The ECHO viruses consist of a ribonucleic acid (RNA) core and a protein coat (capsid) built of numerous subunits (capsomeres). In the mature extracellular virus (virion), the protein coat carries the antigenic specificity and provides a protective shell for the single-stranded ribonucleic acid core which contains the viral genetic material and serves as the essential infectious component. The infectivity of RNA preparations derived from crude cell culture grown ECHO virus types 1 and 8 by the phenol extraction method was first shown by SPRUNT et al. (1959). Such preparations were completely inactivated by RNase but not by DNase and produced plaques on human cell monolayers with the synthesis of complete viral particles. Furthermore, the infectivity of phenol-extracted ribonucleic acid of ECHO virus type 8, for non-primate (rabbit, mouse, guinea pig, chicken, etc.) cultured cells and for animals (mouse, chicken) insusceptible to whole virus is well established (HOLLAND et al., 1959). The result of such *in vitro* and *in vivo* infection was the emergence of complete virions produced in a single cycle of reproduction without any overt CPE or disease. Each virion, thus produced, was found to be identical with the virion from which the infectious RNA was extracted. The infectivity of ECHO virus RNAs for monkey kidney cells can be greatly increased by depleting the cells of calcium and adding to the infectious RNA a facilitator (poorly water soluble compound such as talc and dibasic calcium phosphate dihydrate) which probably serves as a solid vehicle for RNA (ROUHANDEH, 1964). This infectivity, however, is destroyed by snake venom phosphodiesterase (ROUHANDEH and DUBES, 1964). A column chromatography system using hydromagnesite as a facilitator and an increasing phosphate gradient ($0.04\,M - 0.11\,M$) for elution, has been described for the separation of ECHO virus type 7 infectious RNA from cellular RNA. The infectious RNA eluted as a peak at $0.11\,M$ phosphate while the noninfectious cellular portion eluted at the initial low phosphate concentration ($0.04\,M$) (LAMB and DUBES, 1964).

The separation of ECHO virus type 7 RNA from the bulk of cellular (FL cells in which the virus was grown) RNA by column chromatography using methylated albumin columns has been reported (FUKADA and KAWADA, 1963). The cells were infected at a multiplicity of 50 PFU per cell and incubated at 37° C for 3—8 hours. The harvests were suspended in $0.15\,M$ sodium chloride containing 5×10^{-4} methylene-diaminetetraacetic acid and $0.01\,M$ Tris buffer at pH 8.1. The nucleic acid was extracted by the phenol-sodium dodecyl sulfate method at $0-4°$ C and chromatographed at room temperature. The elutes were assayed for infectivity by the plaque method and also examined for ultraviolet absorption. Since the infectivity of viral RNA was found to be uninhibited by cellular RNA at concentrations encountered in such column chromatography, it was concluded that the observed separation was real and that no significant amount of infectious RNA eluted with the cellular RNA.

C. Resistance to Physical and Chemical Agents

The data recounted for properties entered in this subsection relate almost entirely to the intact virus and other extraneous cellular debris into which progeny may be released. At best only crude debris has been removed; the effects these extraneous materials impose, in contrast to "pure" virus, are unknown.

1. Temperature

ECHO viruses are denatured and inactivated at varying rates, depending on environmental factors. The prototypic virus stocks stored at $-70°$ C have been quite stable for periods ranging from 9 months to 4.5 years. But diluted stocks of types 20, 21, and 22 similarly stored may be poorly preserved (KAMITSUKA et al., 1961). Undiluted stocks appear to be preserved as well at $-20°$ C. Inactivation occurs at higher temperatures, probably exponentially. A strain (Haynes) of ECHO virus type 9, suspended in Hanks' saline at pH 7.4—7.8 was incubated for 30 minutes at room temperature, 37°, 45°, 50°, and 55° C. No appreciable loss occurred at room temperature or 37° C (the half-life at this temperature was less than 12 hours), whereas titer reductions of 3 log at 45° C, 4 log at 50° C and apparently complete inactivation at 55° C were observed (TYRRELL et al., 1958). The stability of ECHO virus types 1—20 as undiluted infected cell culture fluids (pH 7.4—7.8) after incubation at 37° C for 2, 4, 8, and 24 hours was studied. Except for type 20 which showed a loss of about 3 log in titer, none was significantly affected under above conditions. When the viruses were diluted 1:10 with maintenance medium containing 2.5% calf serum before incubation at 37° C in order to avoid pH fluctuation, the half-lives of types 1, 4, 6, 9, and 20 in the order mentioned, were found to be 24, 18, 40, 19, and 2.5 hours (LEHMANN-GRUBE and SYVERTON, 1959).

A singular and important property of the ECHO viruses is their stabilization by molar $MgCl_2$ (also molar Ca^{++}) to thermal inactivation at 50° C for 1 to 3 hours (WALLIS and MELNICK, 1962). ECHO virus types 12, 24, and 32 are also stabilized by molar $MgSO_4$ at 50° C. However, other types when suspended in $M\,MgSO_4$ are stabilized (at 50° C) only if subprotective amounts (0.01—0.02 molar) of $MgCl_2$ or NaCl are added (WALLIS et al., 1965). Enteroviruses stabilized with $MgCl_2$ retain full infectivity for at least 3 days at 37° C, for weeks at room temperature, and for some at least a year at 4° C. Monovalent cations (i.e. $2\,M$ Na+) stabilize these viruses at 50° C for only one hour and in contrast to divalent cations, enhance their inactivation at 37° C (WALLIS and MELNICK, 1962).

L-cystine had a variable effect on the stability of ECHO virus types 1, 3, 6, and 19 at 36.5° C and 50° C. At concentrations of 2.5 mg/ml, L-cystine enhanced the inactivation of these viruses when incubated at 36.5° C for 12 hours, whereas 0.5—2.5 mg/ml of L-cystine stabilized ECHO virus type 1 to thermal inactivation at 50° C. Other types were only slightly stabilized under these conditions (POHJANPELTO, 1961). WALLIS and MELNICK (1965a) found only type 4

(Pesascek) among 28 serotypes to be cystine-stabilized against thermal inactivation at 50° C. In addition, this strain differed from the Dutoit strain of the same type in that it required cyst(e)ine in the overlay medium for maximal plaque formation. The results obtained by POHJANPELTO have been attributed (MEL-NICK, 1962) to the effects of HCl and NaOH used to dissolve and neutralize the cystine which, in turn, resulted in the introduction of the monovalent cation Na^+ known to enhance the inactivation of enteroviruses at 37° C and stabilize them at 50° C.

2. Dessication

Several strains of ECHO viruses, namely types 7, 11, and 12 have been dried. Twenty 0.0001 ml drops of infected tissue culture fluid overlays were spread with a microsyringe on glass slides; these dried preparations were stored at 20° C in relative humidities of 20% and 84%. After 2½ hours the slides were washed down with 1 ml of suspended fluid and the suspensions titrated immediately for loss of infectivity. The maximum mean log reduction in titer at relative humidity of 84% was 0.5 logs; the mean log reduction at relative humidity of 20% ranged from 3.7 ("U" strain of type 11) to 1.0 (type 7) $\log_{10}$ (BUCKLAND and TYRRELL, 1962).

3. Photo-inactivation

ECHO viruses (as well as other members of enteroviruses) differ from other groups of viruses in that they are resistant under normal conditions to photo-dynamic inactivation. However, they can be made photo-sensitive to proflavine at pH 9.0—10.0 if they are first cleansed of cell culture organic components by filtration through anion resins. Moreover, photo-sensitization could be achieved when the virus is grown in cell cultures maintained on a simple salt-glucose medium. Under these conditions, ECHO virus types 2, 18, 20, 22, 23, 24, and 30 are completely photosensitized by both toluidine blue and proflavine; types 11, 26, and 32 are completely photosensitized by proflavine but only partially by toluidine blue; type 3 completely by toluidine blue and partially by proflavine and the remaining types are all partially photosensitized by both dyes. The photosensitization effect is reversible; the virus becomes photoresistant when the dye is removed. Lowering the temperature (down to 4° C) or pH (down to 6—7), just before exposure of virus-dye complex to light, also reversed the effect (WALLIS and MELNICK, 1964, 1965b, c). It has been postulated that during irradiation, the virus-dye complex absorbs one photon of light energy and attains metastable excited state. The excited complex then combines with oxygen and thus the infective moiety is rendered inactivated (HIATT et al., 1960).

4. Halogens

The efficiency of chlorine, iodine and bromine as disinfectants in inactivating ECHO viruses in water has been studied by various workers. It is generally agreed that the free halogen is more viricidal than the combined form. Furthermore, the free residual halogen required for inactivation depends on pH, temperature and contact time. The destruction (99%) of ECHO virus type 7 with 10 mg/ml of elemental iodine at 15° C was achieved in 3½ minutes. Under the same conditions, type 9 required about 10 minutes of contact time (KABLER et al., 1961). More recently, ECHO virus types 2 and 9 were diluted in water buffered to pH 7.0—7.7 to give 20—1000 $TCID_{50}$ of virus and the dilutions were mixed with various concentrations of calcium hypochlorite, sodium hypochlorite and iodine in potassium iodide so that the final free halogen concentrations ranged from 2.0 to 0.2 p.p.m. The mixtures were left at room temperature for periods of 1 to 10 minutes, when the halogen was immediately inactivated and the mixtures assayed for virus in cell cultures. The three halogens showed approximately the same viricidal effect after 10 minutes of contact time. Exposure to free chlorine or bromine for one minute required 4 times greater concentration of the agent than exposure for 10 minutes. It was concluded that the presence of 0.5 p.p.m. of free halogen residuals can inactivate virus dosages commonly encountered in swimming pools in 10 minutes (McLEAN, 1963). Some data (BERG et al., 1964) suggest that inactivation of ECHO virus type 7 by elemental iodine was due to the interaction of a single molecule of the halogen on a single vital site of the virus. Polyethoxy-ethanol-iodine (Wescodyne) is an ineffective viricidal agent (exposure time, ≤ 30 minutes) for ECHO virus type 26 and for other enteroviruses (WALLIS et al., 1963).

The functional relationship between rate of inactivation and oxidation potential of ECHO (types 6 and 9) as well as other enteroviruses treated with chloramine T was studied in order to elucidate the reported differences in sensitivity of these viruses to the residual amounts of this halogen. It was found that the same functional relationship exists between rate of inactivation and oxidation potential among these viruses when tested at 37° C and pH 7.0. ECHO virus type 6 was exposed to 1 in 1000 and 0.1 in 1000 dilutions (initial residuals of 150 and 15 p.p.m. respectively) of chloramine T at 37° C. With 150 p.p.m., the oxidation potential measured with a conventional potentiometer was 540 to 560 MV and the activation energy was estimated at 11,600 cal per mol. Type 9 was tested with 1 in 1000 and 0.05 in 1000 (initial residuals of 100—125 and 1 p.p.m. respectively) of chloramine T at a temperature range of 0 to 50° C. Oxidation potentials of 545—570 MV (higher chlorine concentration) and 460—470 MV (lower chlorine concentration) were obtained. In these experiments, the activation energy of oxidation was estimated at 10,300 cal per mol while the activation energy for the spontaneous inactivation at temperatures of 37° to 50° C was estimated at ∼77,500 cal per mol. The data indicated that the two types of ECHO virus and the Coxsackie virus B type 5 and the 3 types of poliovirus which were included in these studies had about the same activation energies for oxidative inactivation and hence equally sensitive to chlorination. Coxsackie virus A type 5, however, was found to be less sensitive to chlorination at temperatures below 37° C (LUND, 1964).

5. Other Chemicals

ECHO viruses are resistant to all known chemotherapeutic agents and antibiotics and are not inactivated by commonly used antiseptics such as 70% ethanol, 5% Lysol and 1% Roccol. They are resistant to ether (20% ethyl ether at 4° C for 18 hours) and deoxycholate. The sensitivity of ECHO virus types 4, 6 and 9 to the analytical reagent grade of chloroform has been investigated.

Mixtures of 0.05 ml of chloroform and 1 ml of infected tissue culture fluids were either shaken by hand at room temperature or in a mechanical mixer at 4° C for 10 minutes. The mixtures were then centrifuged at 400 r.p.m. for 5 minutes and the top clear suspending medium which contained the virus was assayed in cell cultures. All three viruses were found to be resistant to chloroform (FELD-MAN and WANG, 1961).

6. Plant Extracts

The inhibitory activities of 17 plant extracts were tested against ECHO virus types 1—9 and 11—14 in monkey kidney cell cultures. An aqueous extract of the fruiting body of a strain of *Calvatia gigantea* (the giant puffball) had significant inhibitory effects against types 4, 9, and 11 at concentrations of 1:2880, 1:1200 and 1:2880, respectively. The aqueous extract of the residue remaining from ethanol precipitation of the same species had activity against types 7 and 8 at concentrations of 1:960 and 1:920 respectively. The ethanol extraction of the flowers of a species of *Cattleys* showed activity against type 2 at 1:480 concentration. Other extracts were less effective. The antiviral activity was specific and showed the greatest effect when the cell cultures were pretreated with the extract and the virus inoculum did not exceed 100 TCD_{50}. Furthermore, an inhibitory effect on the antibody production in mice by these viruses was also shown for one of the extracts (GOULET et al., 1960).

VI. Antigenic Characteristics

Immunological techniques are important for distinguishing differences in antigenic structure, and for the identification of virus strains. All such uses depend on the immunological specificity of viral antigens. As to the ECHO viruses, knowledge of the antigenic structure of many is incomplete and patchy.

A. Fractionation of Antigens

Infected liquid overlays from monkey kidney cells inoculated with ECHO virus types 12 and 19 have been studied in CsCl equilibrium density gradients in order to determine the distribution of the infectivity, hemagglutinating (HA) and complement-fixing (CF) antigens. With ECHO 19, peak infectivity and 80—90% of HA activity were at a density of 1.34 g/ml. Another peak of HA containing 10—20% of the activity was located at 1.29; the CF antigen was detected at different buoyant densities, ranging from 1.34—1.29. Viral particles with buoyant densities from 1.34 and 1.29 were negatively stained with 1% phosphotungstic acid and studied with the electron microscope. While particles from the former density appeared complete and exhibited a polyhedral structure, those from the latter density were devoid of such a structure and were considered as incomplete particles (FABIYI et al., 1964). Similar results have been obtained with fluid from ECHO virus type 12 infected monkey kidney cells. Two kinds of hemagglutinating particles both showing the characteristic polyhedral structure but one with a buoyant density of 1.33 and representing the complete infectious virus and the other with a density of 1.29 representing the noninfectious empty capsids were observed. Experiments involving ether treatment and heating of the two kinds of particles indicated that the noninfectious particles were less stable (HALPEREN et al., 1964b). None of the evidence thus far obtained indicates a separation of HA or CF antigen from the infectious viral particle (FABIYI and WENNER, 1963).

1. Hemagglutination

Several ECHO viruses agglutinate erythrocytes. GOLDFIELD and colleagues (1957) initially noted agglutination of human type 0 (H—O) red blood cells by types 3, 6, 7, 11, and 12. The specificity of the hemagglutination (HA) was established by inhibition (HI) of homologous antisera. Subsequently types 13, 19, 20, 21, 24, 29, and 30 have been added to the entries (DARDANONI and ZAFFIRO, 1958, 1959; LAHELLE, 1958; PHILIPSON, 1958; ZAFFIRO, 1959; PHILIPSON and ROSEN, 1959; HAMMON et al., 1959; SCHMIDT et al., 1962a; PODOPLEKIN, 1963; GAUDIN et al., 1963; KERN and ROSEN, 1964; BEHBEHANI and WENNER, 1965). Types 3, 7, 11, and 13 grown in human amnion cells while agglutinating human cells failed to have similar effect on sheep, chick and guinea pig erythrocytes. Monkey (presumably *M. mulatta*) erythrocytes may be agglutinated by types 7 (prototype and Genco strain) and 12 (prototype strain only). Red blood cells from other species of monkeys *(Cercopithecus aethiops* and *Erythrocebus patas)* are agglutinable by most hemagglutinating ECHO viruses (GAUDIN et al., 1963).

The HA property appears to be lacking for those ECHO virus serotypes not mentioned above. Moreover strains of the same serotype do not share the HA property equally. The prototype strain (D'Amori) of type 6 does not hemagglutinate; LAHELLE (1958a, b), however, found strains closely related to D'Amori to agglutinate human red cells. While all reports indicate that the ECHO 6 prototype is a nonhemagglutinating virus, varying HA responses have been obtained for strains representing two prototypic prime strains, namely 6' (Cox) and 6" (Burgess) (LAHELLE, 1958b; SCHMIDT et al., 1962a; BUSSELL et al., 1962a; GAUDIN et al., 1963; BEHBEHANI and WENNER, 1965). Similar findings of variation in HA response have been found (KERN and ROSEN, 1964; BEHBEHANI and WENNER, 1965) among strains of types 24 and 30.

Many different factors affect the HA property. The H—O hemagglutinin is stable at −20° C for 2—3 months; some activity is lost when stored at 4° C for a few days, whereas considerable loss occurs on storage at room temperature or at 37° C overnight. Heating at 56° C for a few minutes results in complete loss of HA activity (LAHELLE, 1958a). Maximal titers have been obtained at 37° C and pH 7.0; at least 10^6—10^7 tissue culture infective doses (hereafter referred to as $TCID_{50}$) of virus per ml are required for the production of HA pattern (BUSSELL et al., 1962a). Maximal HA activity is temperature-dependent. KERN and ROSEN (1964) using infant (umbilical cord blood) and adult erythrocytes with various ECHO viruses at 4° and 37° C, found the HA activity to fall into one of 3 categories. Maximal HA titers were obtained for types 3, 11, 13, and 19 and for types 6, 24, 29, and 30 at 4° and 37° C respectively, whereas types 7, 12, 20, and 21 provided similar titers at both temperatures. Newborn (umbilical cord) erythrocytes may be more sensitive indicators of HA (>4- to 8-fold over adult cells), at least for type 13 at 4° C and for type 20 at 37° C. Similar temperature dependencies have been noted by PODOPLEKIN and IVANOVA (1965). Optimal pH values for full HA activity were for type 11, pH 7.4, and for types 20, 21, and 30 (Frater), pH 5.8 (KERN and ROSEN, 1964). A dilute inoculum in combination with a correspondingly delayed development of CPE, and hence late harvest may yield best HA antigen. The infectivity: HA ratios among strains of type 6 which had high infectivity titers (B phase) were 6—7 logs, while those of strains of low infectivity titers (S phase) were ~4—5 logs. Among various strains of ECHO virus type 6, HA production was not correlated with phase, infectivity titer or the level of *in vitro* passage. Heating at 40° C for one hour failed to affect the HA titer, whereas heating at 45° C for one hour caused an 8-fold decrease, while three minutes exposure at 50° C was followed by almost complete loss of HA activity (BUSSELL et al., 1962a). The successive passage of ECHO viruses in cell cultures has not only failed to increase or stabilize the HA property (McINTOSH and SOMMERVILLE, 1959) but may result in de- creased titer (SCHMIDT et al., 1962a; BUSSELL et al., 1962a) or with stable cell cultures (HeLa, KB, HEp-2 and stable monkey kidney) in loss of the HA property (MAISEL et al., 1961; PODOPLEKIN, 1964). The receptor substances on human red cells have been purified (100 ×) and analyzed chemically. The purified material was composed of about 31% lipid, 60% protein and 9% carbohydrates; had a buoyant density of 1.18, and a S20°, w of 14 Svedberg units. A deoxypolynucleo- tide, containing adenine, thymine, cytosine and guanine is firmly attached to the receptor structure (PHILIPSON et al., 1964). That both complete and in- complete viral particles, which are produced during the growth of ECHO virus types 12 and 19 in cell culture, are capable of agglutinating erythrocytes has been well established (HALPEREN et al., 1964b; FABIYI et al., 1964).

Attachment of virus to erythrocyte receptor involves two stages: the first, reversible by chymotrypsin, shows no, or little temperature dependence, and has a pH optimum of 5.5; the second develops as a progressive resistance to chymotrypsin, with a pH optimum above 8, and appears to be temperature dependent (PHILIPSON and BENGTSSON, 1962). Later studies (PHILIPSON and LIND, 1964) on the interaction between the purified receptor substance and purified P^{32} labeled ECHO virus type 7 also involved two stages. The second stage was irreversible, had a sharp optimum pH of 7.6 and followed first-order kinetics, and thus was assumed to be enzymatic. Furthermore, the reaction caused the release of high molecular weight RNase-susceptible infectious RNA. As noted earlier certain mercaptide-forming sulfhydryl reagents, such as p-chloro- mercuribenzoate (PCMB) can react with the sulfhydryl groups on a hemag- glutinating ECHO virus, and thus interfere with viral hemagglutination. This inactivation of viral HA activity can be reversed by thiol compounds (i.e. reduced glutathione) (PHILIPSON and CHOPPIN, 1960). More than 97% inactivation of the HA property, and 6.5-fold reduction in PFU of ECHO virus type 7 have been produced by $10^{-4} M$ of 2,3-dimercaptopropanol (BAL). The activity of this compound was attributed to its oxidized product (a polymer containing disulfide bonds) which formed a mixed disulfide with virus — SH groups, thereby blocking adsorption to receptors. It should be pointed out that the reduced form of BAL is a dithiol belonging to the thiol compounds which, as referred to above, can reactivate the inactivated viruses. BAL-inactivated virus could be reactivated by mercaptoethanol but not by agents which split thiol esters (PHILIPSON and CHOPPIN, 1962).

ECHO virus type 7 does not seem to destroy the receptors on erythrocytes during hemagglutination, and thus the cells remain agglutinable by another virus belonging to the same type or another, such as type 11 (GAUDIN et al., 1963). Following hemagglutination, types 3, 11, 12, and certain strains of types 20 and 25 could be eluted from the human erythrocytes (at 37° C within 4—6 hours) while serotypes 6, 7, 13, 19, and some strains of 20 and 25 could not be eluted at various temperatures (4°, 22°, and 37° C). Red cells from which the virus was eluted were still agglutinable by the same or another serotype. The agglutinability of erythrocytes was destroyed by trypsin and formalin, while RDE or potassium periodate showed no such effect (PODOPLEKIN, 1964).

HA inhibitors may be found in infected and noninfected cell cultures. Inhibitors associated with cell cultures fall into two categories, namely, 1) those derived apparently from the specific receptors of human red cells and intact HeLa cells as well as certain subcellular fractions thereof, and 2) as yet unspecified constituents apparently unrelated to cell receptors (PHILIPSON and BENGTSSON, 1962; SCHMIDT et al., 1964a). The latter are called tissue culture (TC) inhibitors, and are found in infected and uninfected HeLa, and also in non-primate cell (e.g. hamster kidney) culture fluids. TC inhibitors are distinguished from receptor inhibitors by several characteristics, such as stability at 60° C for 30 minutes, inactivation by genetron, ether and other organic solvents, and their occurrence in cell culture fluids rather than cell homogenates. Both types of inhibitors are considered to be lipoprotein in nature. Receptor inhibitors are destroyed by proteolytic enzymes.

Most human and animal sera contain nonspecific inhibitors which can affect HA of intratypic strains of ECHO viruses in differing degrees. PODOPLEKIN and IVANOVA (1965) noted three levels of sensitivity, namely low, medium and high, which corresponded to ≤4-, 8- to 16- and ≥32-fold decrease in HA titer. No correlation was found between serum inhibitor-sensitivity and temperature-dependency. Serum inhibitors are heat stable and resistant to treatment with RDE, periodate, organic solvents (genetron, ether, chloroform, acetone), protein denaturing agents (phenol, formaldehyde) and individual proteolytic and lipolytic enzymes. However, a combination of chymotrypsin and phospholipase destroyed such inhibitors, indicating that serum inhibitors are structured within a phospholipid-protein complex (SCHMIDT et al., 1964b). These inhibitors have also been satisfactorily removed by adsorption with 0.1% bentonite and by treatment with filtrates of a psychrophilic Pseudomonas species (BUSSELL et al., 1962a; SCHMIDT et al., 1964c).

2. Complement Fixation

ECHO viruses provide reliable antigens for use in empirical CF tests and have been helpful in defining serological specificity, or the existence of cross-relationships between heterotypic enteroviruses. The preparation in infected tissue cultures of antigens of satisfactory potency and specificity is based largely on the poliomyelitis model (SCHMIDT et al., 1957) where the factors favoring optimal yields include a large host cell population, low concentration of serum in the medium, and harvest when CPE is maximal. In contrast with the numerous studies on the nature of poliovirus CF antigens (MAYER et al., 1957; LENNETTE et al., 1964) similar information has not yet become available for the ECHO viruses.

In some early studies, ARCHETTI et al. (1957) noted that untreated ECHO virus infected monkey kidney tissue culture cells often yielded unsatisfactory CF antigens with antisera prepared in monkeys. Types 1—3 and 5—13 were adapted to HeLa cells; infected fluids from the fifth passage in these cells provided specific reliable antigens for use in the CF test. Later work showed that fluid overlays derived from infected monkey kidney cells maintained in lactalbumin hydrolysate medium containing calf serum were, after treatment with fluorocarbon, useful CF antigens, giving no or slight cell-culture antigen-antibody reactions thereto, and thereby revealing type-specific responses (HALONEN et al., 1958a, b). With both HeLa and purified monkey kidney antigens, reciprocal crosses were obtained between types 1, 8, and 13, and a one-way cross between type 13 antigen and type 12 antiserum. These cross reactions have been observed also by serum neutralization (and, as was shown later [HAMMON et al., 1959a] due to a mixture of type 1 and 13 viruses).

The handicaps relating to nonspecific reactions have been serious obstacles in definitive studies on antigenic relationships. A major handicap has been the emergence of antibodies to non-viral protein present in the infected tissue culture fluid overlay. An attempt was made to prepare specific ECHO virus antisera without interfering host CF antibodies; monkey kidney cell culture grown antigens were treated with fluorocarbon prior to inoculation of guinea pigs. Of twelve treated antigens which did not possess any host-antigen CF activity, nine induced satisfactory antisera with no host-CF antibodies, and three induced antisera which possessed host-antibodies, but titers of the latter were 16—32 times lower than the specific viral antibodies. Another approach to the same problem was made by growing ECHO virus type 4 in Detroit-504 human fibroblast-like cells; the infected fluid after treatment with fluorocarbon and concentration was emulsified in Arlacel-Bayol F adjuvant prior to injection into guinea pigs and monkeys. The antisera thus produced were highly specific and did not react nonspecifically with fluorocarbon treated CF antigen derived from monkey kidney cells (YOHN and HAMMON, 1960). SHINGU (1961) on studying the effect of heating (56° C—85° C for 30 minutes) on the CF antigens of ECHO viruses found that the antigenic potency of ECHO virus types 1, 3, 7, 8, 11, 12, 13, 14, 15, 16, 17, and 18 was either unchanged, or lower after heat treatment (designated CFt—), while that of types 2, 5, 6, and 9 was enhanced after such treatment (designated CFt+).

3. Serum Neutralization

The prototype ECHO viruses after many passages in susceptible cell cultures provide high yields of virus ($\sim 10^6$ TCID$_{50}$) which behave fairly predictably in conventional serum-neutralization tests. On the other hand, it is quite clear that fresh isolates (e.g. types 4, 6, 30, etc.) may be poorly neutralized by prototypic antisera. BARRON and KARZON (1965) have pointed out for type 6 the existence of variant forms (see section on antigenic variation) one of which is poorly neutralized by homologous antisera. CHOPPIN and EGGERS (1962) working with a strain of Coxsackie virus B4 isolated two kinds of virus particles; one forms small plaques which is much more sensitive to specific antibody than the other which forms large plaques. Others have encountered early virus "break-through" with homotypic strains suggesting differing sensitivities of homotypes to specific antibody. Thus far published accounts of separating and characterizing intratypic ECHO virus variants relate largely to type 6.

Plaque development is reduced by specific antibody (see cytotoxic sera, above) and is the basis for plaque reduction (WENNER et al., 1959) or plaque inhibition tests (SAKURADA and PRINCE, 1961). Within limits of virus input the dose-response curve is essentially linear. With the disc method (inhibition of plaque formation by antiserum impregnated filter paper discs) there is a linear relationship between the log of the antiserum dilution and the diameter of the inhibition zone. Apparently more sensitive, and able to maintain a more enduring equilibrium state than serum-virus union in tube cultures, the method has found application in intratypic strain differentiation (based on differing rates of neutralization) and in revealing antibodies (e.g. type 4) that may be masked in the less sensitive tube culture system.

4. Other Methods
a) Labeled Antigens

As noted earlier, antigen developed in infected cell cultures may be revealed by fluorescence microscopy. Antibody conjugated with fluorescein isothiocyanate is absorbed to remove nonspecific fluorescence, and then applied to infected cell sheets; such cells would show fluorescence mainly in the cytoplasm. The method using either single or pooled antisera (SHAW et al., 1961) has not found wide application in diagnosis. Both direct and indirect methods have been used to measure antibody responses in individuals infected with type 9 (RIGGS et al., 1962). For a recent review see CHEEVER (1964).

b) Precipitins

A micro-precipitin gel diffusion method was used to detect specific ECHO virus antigens in cell cultures, and for measurement of specific antibody response in man. High virus concentrations (10^7 $TCID_{50}$ per 0.1 ml) but only 0.015 ml of serum were required for obtaining reliable results. Reciprocal precipitation of ECHO virus types 1 and 8 was obtained with hyperimmune sera prepared against each (MIDDLETON et al., 1964).

B. Antigenic Variations
1. Type Specific Antisera

The identity of enterovirus serotypes is based on their serological specificities. Following naturally-occurring infections with specific serotypes, or after inoculation of the serotypes into animals, specific humoral antibodies develop. The major difficulty encountered with human sera relates not to their specificity, but often to their cross-reactivity with other serotypes. On the other hand, animals inoculated with purified virus stocks provide type-specific antisera, not only useful for both within and between serotypes. The production of specific antisera for the first 25 prototypic ECHO viruses in rhesus and cynomolgus monkeys and their standardization have been described (KAMITSUKA et al., 1961). Monkeys were inoculated by the intramuscular route with mixtures of equal amounts of un-diluted virus and mineral oil adjuvant. The antisera thus produced were type-specific, and with the exception of ECHO virus types 4 and 21, all others had high serum dilution endpoints. Satisfactory antisera have been produced in rabbits by intramuscular and intravenous inoculation of virus-adjuvant mixtures, and in guinea pigs inoculated subcutaneously and intracardially, or intraperi-toneally with fluorocarbon treated virus (Microbiological Associates, 1957; HALONEN and HUEBNER, 1960). ECHO viruses concentrated (to one-tenth the original volume) by precipitation with $25\,mM$ $AlCl_3$ and $50\,mM$ Na_2CO_3 and treated at 50° C in $M\,MgCl_2$ to eliminate several undesired agents (e.g. SV_{40} and PPLO), have produced very good antibody responses, especially in guinea pigs and large animals (horses, cows, sheep, goats, pigs and baboons). Such con-centrated antigens, except ECHO virus type 4, produced high-titer (1:1000 to 1:20,000) antisera in horses and in baboons (MELNICK et al., 1964; MIDULLA et al., 1965; OCAMPO and MELNICK, 1964).

Identification of enterovirus isolates may be quickened using combination patterns so designed that each serum is included in more than one pool (LIM and BENYESH-MELNICK, 1960; SCHMIDT et al., 1961). Identification is confirmed by retest of isolates against the single serum shared by the pools.

a) Crosses Obtained with Animal Antisera

ECHO virus type 8 shares antigens with ECHO virus type 1, the latter having the broader spectrum. The extent of crossing between ECHO virus types 1 and 8 in both serum neutralization and CF tests is so marked that differentiation is difficult. Reciprocal precipitins have been found by gel diffusion (MIDDLETON et al., 1964). Similar cross-reactivity was not observed by fluorescence antibody labeling (SHAW et al., 1961). In addition to these crosses, antisera of both types 1 and 8 cross react in neutralization and CF tests with ECHO 12. On the other hand, neutralization titers with type 12 antisera are low for types 1 and 8 (COMMITTEE ON ENTEROVIRUSES, 1957; KAMITSUKA et al., 1961; BERG et al., 1962). The cross between types 1 and 13 viruses was due to contamination of type 13 with type 1 (HAMMON et al., 1959a); a similar situation applied to the crossings obtained for types 29 and 30 (SCHMIDT et al., 1964d; ROSEN et al., 1965). In a study of antigenic relationships between strains of ECHO virus types 6 and 30 (BEHBEHANI and WENNER, 1965) significant antigenic relationship be-tween the heterotypes was not detected by serum neutralization or HI; however, significant one-way crosses were obtained in CF tests with type 6 antisera and type 30 antigens. Several other reciprocal crosses have been noted, namely between types 22, 23 and 24 by CF (WIGAND and SABIN, 1961) and between type 22 virus and type 23 antisera by serum neutralization. Minor reciprocal neutralization has been obtained for types 11 and 19 (KAMITSUKA et al., 1961). Using rabbit antiserum, LAHELLE (1958b) observed a one-way cross between these latter types; he also noted reciprocal crossing between types 3 and 13.

b) Crosses Encountered with Human Sera

Infection of human beings with several enteroviruses may evoke heterotypic serological responses. Such responses have been obtained more often by CF than by serum neutralization. The following accounts illustrate some of the findings. CF antibodies for ECHO virus types 6 and 9 followed infection with type 4 (JOHNSSON et al., 1958a). A distinctive rise in antibodies for type 16 has been noted (NEVA and MALONE, 1959a) following human infection with ECHO virus types 6, 9 and 20, and Coxsackie virus group B, type 3. SCHMIDT et al. (1962c) obtained heterotypic CF responses to ECHO types 12 and 19 among patients infected with types 4, 6, 9 and 11 ECHO viruses. A striking complex of heterotypic responses was obtained by HALONEN et al. (1959) following natural or experimental infection with ECHO 16 and 20, polio-type 1, and Coxsackie B3 viruses. While the antibody response varied, many responded to heterotypic ECHO (types 2, 4, 5, 6, 7, 8, 11 and 20) and Coxsackie viruses (group B, types 1, 3, 4 and 5). Antibodies for poliovirus type 1 were obtained after type 6 (VON ZEIPEL and SVEDMYR, 1957) and type 9 (LENNETTE et al., 1961) ECHO virus infections. Similar serological responses for group B Coxsackie viruses attended infections with ECHO viruses types 4, 6, 9, 16 and 20 (JOHNSSON et al., 1958b; BERGLUND et al., 1958).

The antigenic relationships demonstrable by complement fixation are intertwined with differences in methodologies making interpretations exceedingly difficult. For example, in studies noted above CF antigens were either heat-inactivated or treated with fluorocarbon. In addition to those noted, antibodies for polioviruses using heat-inactivated antigen have been found among patients infected with Coxsackie and ECHO viruses (HAMMON et al., 1958). In another study using untreated poliovirus antigens, only a small fraction (22 of 579) of individuals with laboratory evidence of non-poliovirus infections developed antibodies to polioviruses. Many of these cross reactions were obtained among patients with ECHO virus type 9 infections suggesting that polioviruses and ECHO virus type 9 share common antigens (LENNETTE et al., 1961). In yet another study using untreated antigens, cross reactions obtained between types 4, 6 and 9 might indicate cross-relationship, excepting that the clinical circumstances strongly suggested that all might be related to recently acquired infections (BUSSELL et al., 1962b). Despite all these crosses with human sera, suggesting striking antigenic overlaps among enteroviruses, freshly isolated strains (untreated) can often be identified by CF using known antisera prepared in animals (GODFREDSON, 1960; GNESH et al., 1964).

Similar cross reactions have been encountered less frequently in HI tests. In the studies of BUSSELL et al. (1962b), 2 of 15 patients infected with type 6 had titer increases to type 12. A corresponding increase in serum neutralizing antibodies was not found. Infections with ECHO virus types 4 and 9 have been followed by rises in HI antibodies to ECHO virus type 6.

The few heterologous antibody responses obtained in serum neutralization tests relate to serotypes already mentioned. By and large the extensive crossings noted by CF have not been found by serum neutralization, and the few described may well relate to recent infection with the heterotype. KRECH (1957) noted serological cross neutralization between ECHO type 9 and herpes simplex viruses. This has not been confirmed (MELNICK, 1958).

Despite an extensive serologic overlap between types, the nature of the antigen(s) responsible for the heterologous antibody has not been elucidated. While a large body of evidence suggests that enterovirus heterotypes may share similar antigens, the evidence is largely associative.

c) Variation within Serotypes

Intratypic variants exist for many of the serotypes. These strains differ from one another and from the prototype in various characteristics (e.g. type 16) (NEVA et al., 1959). A strain may differ by being poorly neutralized by antiserum against the prototype, and yet is capable of producing antibody with broad capacity to neutralize itself and the prototype. This characteristic is well illustrated by the two variants (prime strains) of prototype ECHO virus type 6 (D'Amori), namely ECHO virus 6' (Cox) and ECHO virus 6'' (Burgess) (Committee on Enteroviruses, 1957; MELNICK, 1957). Somewhat later, newly isolated type 6 strains obtained during an epidemic of aseptic meningitis were found to show considerable serologic variation (KARZON et al., 1959; BARRON and KARZON, 1965; SUTO et al., 1965a, 1965b). Strains recently isolated in primary MK cells were designated "S phase" or "low passage" virus, whereas variants appearing after multiple passage in cell culture were designated "B phase" or "high passage" virus. S phase viruses were poorly neutralized by homologous antiserum, were weakly cytopathic and attained low infectivity titers. In comparison, B phase viruses were readily neutralized, showed fast CPE and yielded high infectivity titers. Further analyses indicated that the two variants consisted of populations of two mutants each with distinguishable characteristics. Virus populations recoverable from the human alimentary tract were predominantly M^+ (large plaque) mutants and possessed the three properties mentioned above for the low passage or S phase viruses. However, on repeated passage in monkey kidney cells the predominant M^+ virus changed to M (minute plaque) mutants which now possessed the characteristics of high passage or B phase viruses. Upon inoculation of monkey kidney cells with artificial mixtures of the two mutants, the yield of M virus per cell was 30- to 1000-fold greater than the yield of M^+ virus. However, in certain human cells, i.e. AV_3, the yield of M^+ virus was 30- to 300-fold greater than in monkey kidney cells. Additionally, the development of minute plaques by M mutants was related to the presence of inhibitors in agar; the latter effect was readily nullified by the addition of polybasic compound protamine to the agar overlay. The predominance of M^+ virus in the human intestinal tract was postulated to be due to the preferential growth of M^+ mutant in human cells, and also, perhaps, to inhibition of M mutant by naturally occurring polyanions (e.g. heparin).

Serologic variations have been encountered also among type 4 ECHO viruses. The prototype (Pesascek) strain isolated by MELNICK (1954) is poorly neutralized by homologous antisera using the tube test. However, as stated earlier, the same antisera gave a plaque reduction titer of ~1:2000 (Committee on Entero-viruses, 1957) indicating the impotence of the antigen. Serological studies on sera obtained from patients with aseptic meningitis provided additional evidence of disparity of strains in measuring antibody rises (CHIN et al., 1957; MALHERBE et al., 1957).

The weak capacity of the type 4 prototype antiserum to neutralize the homo-type was not due to dissociation of virus-antibody complex. Neutralizing antibody-combining tests, using either live or inactivated virus, showed that the Pesascek serum was bound to the Pesascek virus as firmly as to the Dutoit virus (MAL-HERBE et al., 1957), but did not render the prototype virus noninfective. While both the prototype virus and the prototype serum passed through a $0.220\,\mu$ millipore filter the infective virus-antibody complex was retained (WALLIS et al., 1965d).

BARRON and KARZON (1961) compared strains recovered from a local epidemic (Buffalo, N.Y.) with strains isolated in the U.S.A. and S. Africa, including the prototype. All strains were identifiable using antisera prepared in monkeys against strains Shropshire (Buffalo) or Pesascek (the prototype); the Buffalo strains by tube test were antigenically closer to Dutoit than to the prototype. Such distinctions were not readily revealed by plaque reduction. In cross-tests using antisera prepared in rabbits against these and other strains, there was such a great intratypic variation in titer ratios that classification of strains would be exceedingly difficult (BARRON and KARZON, 1961).

The Dutoit strain isolated in S. Africa is a sensitive indicator for measurement of neutralizing antibodies, as is another designated 5705 (YOHN et al., 1960). Just why Dutoit should be better than many others for detection of antibodies in tube tests is not fully understood. The prototype and Dutoit strains are scarcely distinguishable as regards the course and sequence of viral antigen formation *in vitro*, using acridine orange and fluorescence antibody staining to study intra-cellular development (JAMISON et al., 1963). With Dutoit, an increase in cyto-plasmic RNA was detectable two hours earlier than with Pesascek. The buoyant density of both viruses in cesium chloride was 1:35; viral particles of both were morphologically identical by electron microscopy. Differences in cystine-depen-dence and chromatographic behavior have been noted earlier. The $TCID_{50}$ values of Dutoit exceed those of other homotypes. Serum "break-through" is less pronounced with Dutoit than others. The suggestion has been made that Dutoit resembles the B phase of type 6 viruses, whereas other resemble those of the S phase. But conversion of strain Shropshire from the S to B phase has not been reported. In practice the Dutoit strain has been a more satisfactory anti-gen in tube tests for detecting neutralizing antibodies in human sera; other strains (e.g. Pesascek and Shropshire) may be used in plaque reduction tests. Similar variations, less extensive in magnitude have been noted between strains in the CF test (YOHN et al., 1960).

Intratypic strains of types 30 and 31, like the ECHO 6 viruses, differ from one another in the HA property, and often vary strikingly with respect to neutraliza-tion by homotypic antisera (WENNER et al., 1963; BEHBEHANI and WENNER, 1965; BEHBEHANI et al., in preparation).

VII. Interactions with Man and Other Mammalian Species

A. Clinical Expressions

1. The Central Nervous System

ECHO viruses have found clinical expression chiefly in injury of the central nervous system (CNS). The major clinical manifestation has been that of benign lymphocytic meningitis, usually uncomplicated but occasionally associated with encephalitis, bulbo-spinal or spinal paralysis. Minor clinical expressions, occurring both in patients with or without meningitis may involve either the cutaneous,

Table 4. *ECHO Viruses Associated with Human Disease*

Serotype	Nervous system						Other systems					
		Paralysis		Encephalitis					Respiratory			
	Meningitis	Spinal	Bulbospinal	Brain	Cerebellum	Peripheral neuropathies	Skin rash	Gastrointestinal	Upper resp. infection	Pleurodynia	Orchitis	Other
1	+	P					P		+			
2	+	+	+	?			P+	P	+	P		
3	+		?	P			P		+			mild, febrile carditis ?
4	+	+	+	P			+		+			mesenteric adenitis ?
5	+						P	P				febrile
6	+	+		+		?	P	P	+			
7	+	P+		P			P	P	P			
8	+							P	P	P		
9	+	P+	P	P	P	?	+		+	P	P	carditis ?
11	+	P	P				P	P+	+			
12	P						P	?				
13	+	P										
14	+	P+		P			P	P+				
15	+											
16	+	P					+		+			
17	+											
18	+	P		P			P	+				fatal
19	+			P			P	P	P			
20	+						P1	P	P			
21	+											
22	P+					?		P	P			
23	+							P				
24	−							P				
25	+								P			febrile
26	−											none ?
27	+											none ?
29	−											febrile ?
30	+	+	P	+								
31	+	P										
32												
33	−											

+, definite association; P, presumptive association; 1 enanthema; −, no available data.

gastro-intestinal and/or respiratory systems. Occasionally cerebellar ataxia, peripheral neuropathies, hepato-renal dysfunction, orchitis, pleurodynia or carditis may intervene during infections involving several serotypes (Table 4).

a) Benign Lymphocytic Meningitis

WALLGREN (1924) proposed the term benign meningitis to define a nosological clinical entity characterized by fever, headache, nuchal rigidity and lymphocytic pleocytosis. Lethargy, irritability and vomiting are frequently found in young children. Recurrent epidemics of benign meningitis have been associated with types 4, 6, 9, and 30. Clusters of meningitis cases, very likely representing the major clinical expressions of a much wider infection rate have been noted for types 5, 7, 14, 25, and 31. Of the 31 serotypes, according to our information only 6 have *not* been associated with the meningitis syndrome (Table 4).

b) Meningoencephalomyelitis

Brain stem. ECHO viruses may produce disease mimicking bulbo-spinal polio-myelitis (STEIGMAN, 1958; VERLINDE and WILTERDINK, 1958; STEIGMAN and LIPTON, 1960). ECHO virus types 2 and 9 have been isolated from human CNS tissues; type 11 was involved on the basis of virus in feces and attendant antibody rise. The production of experimental poliomyelitis in monkeys with the CNS tissues of the infant presumably succumbing to type 9 was traced subsequently to the concomittant presence of poliovirus type 2 (VERLINDE et al., 1961; PETTE et al., 1961). A corresponding situation does not, apparently, apply to type 11 wherein poliovirus antibodies were not found, but could apply to type 2, where polioviruses might have been eclipsed during an 18-day survival period.

Facial palsies and encephalitis have been encountered during epidemics of types 9 and 30 (SABIN et al., 1958; LANDSMAN et al., 1961). ARCHETTI et al. (1956) listed meningoradiculitis as a clinical feature; they also described patients developing the Guillain-Barré syndrome. The linkage of some of these illnesses with type 9 virus is circumstantial.

Acute cerebellar ataxia, associated with staggering gait, intention tremors, hypotonia, dysarthria, dysmetria, and nystagmus has been encountered with type 9 (McALLISTER et al., 1959), as well as with polio- and Coxsackie viruses. In the Milwaukee outbreak (1957) among 213 patients hospitalized with benign aseptic meningitis, signs of more extensive involvement of the CNS developed in 6 virologically proved instances. Of the 6, 4 had involvement of vestibular nuclei, 1 had evidence of 10th cranial nerve involvement and 1 had transient myelitis. Ataxia and nystagmus were noted in 2 of the 5 with signs indicating brain-stem involvement. Infections with types 6 and 30 have provided clinical evidence of similar penetration into the CNS.

Muscle weakness and paralysis. Limb paralysis simulating paralytic polio-myelitis may develop during infection with several serotypes. BUSER et al. (1957) recovered type 4 virus from a 32-year-old woman with bilateral limb para-lysis. Others (SABIN et al., 1958; FOLEY et al., 1959; PLAGER and HARRISON, 1961; REINHARDT, 1963) have reported similar episodes in children and adults for types 9 and 14. During an outbreak in Minnesota (KLEINMAN et al., 1964) about 5% of the group with CNS disease from ECHO 30 developed limb and truncal paralysis. Similar clinical associations during ECHO 30 infections were noted elsewhere (LANDSMAN et al., 1961; LENNETTE et al., 1962).

Muscular dysfunction of lesser severity however is the rule, chiefly involving neck, trunk and girdle muscles. Type 6 should be added to those listed above (KARZON et al., 1956; KIBRICK et al., 1957); these serotypes have been associated with varying degrees of disability. Types 2, 7, 11, 14, and 16 very likely provoke similar affects (HAMMON et al., 1958; GRIST and BELL, 1963). Muscular disability is seldom permanent; lost reflexes are restored and muscle strength is regained in the ensuing weeks of convalescence. Persistent limb weakness has been reported (PLAGER et al., 1961). KING and KARZON (1962) in a follow-up of 93 persons 3 years after type 6 CNS infection found none with gross evidence of neuromuscular dysfunction; subtle marginal neurological aberrations in both patient and control groups were noted. Minor disorders of behavior, easy fatigability, headache and subjective weakness of back and legs appeared to be related to their earlier illness. Others have also called attention to the importance of ECHO and Coxsackie viruses in the etiology of transient muscular dysfunction (WEHRLE et al., 1959; LEPOW et al., 1962).

2. The Skin and Mucous Membranes

Rashes indistinguishable from exanthem subitum, rubella or meningococcemia occur during infection with several ECHO viruses. The lesions are most often macular or maculopapular; less often they are vesicular. The nature of the cutaneous response requires critical study, to wit, whether primarily a direct viral effect, an antigen-antibody reaction (hypersensitivity) or occasionally related to medicinals used in therapy. Cytopathology of cutaneous lesions has yet to be described.

Of the 31 serotypes 13 have been associated with rashes. Types 9 and 16 have an unmistakable association with disease; types 2, 4, 6, and 11, and perhaps others listed in Table 4 probably involve the skin in expression of clinical pathology. Of all only type 11 has been isolated directly from cutaneous lesions (CHERRY et al., 1963).

To provide a reader with the protean features of the clinical response a summary of the cutaneous eruptions associated with types 4, 9, and 16 follows:

ECHO 4: JOHNSSON et al. (1958a) described a fine blotchy efflorescence localized to the face, and less often to trunk, arms and legs, usually appearing during the first and third days of illness, but occasionally developing during the second bout of a biphasic febrile course. Both FORBES (1958) and KARZON et al. (1961) reported similar findings. During 1964, in Kentucky (RAY et al., 1966). 13 per cent of children with aseptic meningitis, and 10 per cent of those with minor illness developed a rubelliform rash during the later part of the epidemic. Occurring 1 to 3 days after onset of illness it disappeared within 24 to 48 hours. Erythematous, macular and non-pruritic, the rash appeared first on the trunk, occasionally on the face, then became semiconfluent spreading to the extremities. It should be noted that others (LEHAN et al., 1957; MALHERBE et al., 1957; WILSEN et al., 1961) have not encountered skin rashes in circumscribed outbreaks.

ECHO 9: Cutaneous lesions were not reported as a feature of the Italian outbreak (ARCHETTI et al., 1956), or of the earliest outbreaks in Great Britain; such lesions were commonly encountered however, in a fraction of persons attacked during outbreaks occurring later in Europe, Great Britain, Iceland, North America and Australia.

Infants and young children are prime subjects; the highest incidence of rash in Milwaukee was in children less than 3 years of age. The rash usually appears within a day or two after onset of illness. Generally it is maculo-papular (1 to 3 mm in dia-meter), of brown (CRAWFORD et al., 1956) or pink hue, involving the face, trunk and extensor surfaces of the limbs as well as the palms and soles. Among 43 persons from whom virus was recovered in Milwaukee, the rash generally appeared first on the face, or face and neck; spread to other parts of the body occurred within 6 to 12 hours. The rash was confined to the face in 25 per cent, to the face and neck in 11 per cent, to the face, neck and chest in 8 per cent; face, trunk and extremities were all involved in 56 per cent of the patients. Petechiae and ecchymoses may resemble the cutaneous lesions of meningococcemia (FROTHINGHAM, 1958). An enanthema characterized by white or grayish "spots" may develop on the buccal mucosa opposite the molar teeth (TYRRELL and SNELL, 1956; SABIN et al., 1958); small vesicles and ulcers may also appear on the tongue (HORSTMANN, 1958). Biphasic, and rarely triphasic febrile cour-ses occur, each with recrudescence of rash. All signs previously mentioned may not be seen in the same patient. Illness encompasses meningitis without rash, rash without meningitis (at least occult), meningitis with rash, and abortive forms sometimes referred to as "summer grippe".

ECHO 16 (The Boston Exanthema): During the summer of 1951 more than 2000 children in Massachusetts developed mild illnesses associated with skin eruptions (NEVA et al., 1954). A similar but less extensive outbreak of the same disease occurred in Pittsburgh, Pennsylvania (USA) in 1954 (NEVA, 1956). Viruses were recovered (NEVA and ENDERS, 1954) which were closely related to others recovered from patients with aseptic meningitis (KIBRICK et al., 1957). One of the latter strains (Harrington) is the prototype of ECHO 16.

Other signs of illness precede the rash. These include fever (100—102° F), sore throat, headache, shaking chills, myalgia and burning or pain in the eyes. Such signs are more prominent in adults than children. In children, fever and other symptoms last but a day or two; in adults they persist for several more days. As a rule the rash appears several days after onset of illness, and often within a day or two after subsi-dence of fever. It is macular, salmon-pink, sometimes blotchy, resembling the exan-thema of rubella. Macules, measuring 1 to 2 mm in diameter are usually discrete, sometimes scanty, otherwise pronounced and occasionally confluent. Most prominent on the face, neck and trunk, occasionally the rash involves the extremities and palms and soles. Enanthema, consisting of vesicles and shallow ulcers on the mucous mem-branes of the throat, gingival margins and buccal mucosa were noted in Boston, but not in Pittsburgh.

The rash was much more common in children than in adults. Multiple cases occurred simultaneously in families. During the 1954 outbreak in Pittsburgh 32 per cent of the households, 24 per cent of the children and 10 per cent of the adults in one circumscribed community were affected during a 12-day period. The incubation period ranged from 3 to 8 days (NEVA, 1956).

Other serotypes have been associated with skin rashes; these include type 2 (RENDTORFF et al., 1964), type 3 (JORDAN, 1959), type 5 (SELWYN and HOWITT, 1962), type 6 (KARZON et al., 1962), type 7 (BELL et al., 1963), type 8 (SABIN et al., 1958), type 11 (CHERRY et al., 1963), type 14 (SABIN et al., 1958), type 18 (MEDEARIS and KRAMER, 1959), type 19 (CRAMBLETT et al., 1962) and type 20 (CLARKE and STOTT, 1961). Buccal lesions not unlike Koplik's spots were seen in type 20 infections. The rubella-like papular rash described for type 2 re-sembled that seen in type 9 disease.

When met with sporadically, clinical differentiation of rashes etiologically related to ECHO viruses is perplexing, not only between enteroviruses but other exanthema also. The clinical characteristics of rashes are not often helpful in identification; indeed the overlapping signs simply add to the woes of the perplexed clinician! Moreover it would not be unkind to say that in a number of instances the union between these viruses and cutaneous lesions is still one of questionable legitimacy.

3. The Alimentary Tract

Despite the frequency of acute gastroenteritis the etiologic agents responsible for sporadic and epidemic illnesses have largely been undefined. Recently several specific ECHO viruses have been recovered during isolated outbreaks. EICHENWALD et al. (1958) identified type 18 among premature and full-term infants during a mild outbreak of enteritis. LEPINE et al. (1960) found similar association for type 14. Gastroenteritis in adults (BUCKLAND et al., 1959; KLEIN et al.,

Table 5. *Enteroviruses and Infantile Diarrhea*

Locale	Time		Age of patients (years)	No. patients	% yielding enteroviruses		Incidence of enteroviruses ratio Patients/ Controls
	Year	Season(s)			Patients	Controls	
Cincinnati	1955—1956	Summer	0—4	153	48-50	20	6:1 (1956)
Glasgow	1957	All	0—5	338	19	14	2—3:1
Montreal	1958—1959	All	Pediatric age-group	74	8	3	—
Toronto	1959—1960	5 outbreaks	0—2	208	0	6.4	—
Toronto	1960—1961	3 outbreaks	infants	80	2.5	3.6	—
Houston	1959—1961	All	0—2	390	5.6	4.4	1.5:1
Mexico City	1960	Summer-Fall	0—5	404[1]	49.0	10.0	3.9:1

From a table by Yow et al., Amer. J. Hyg. 77, 283 (1963) with additions.

[1] Figures for enteroviruses only, assuming most unidentified agents are enteroviruses.

References:
RAMOS-ALVAREZ and SABIN: J. Amer. med. Ass. 167, 147 (1958).
SOMMERVILLE: Lancet 2, 1347 (1958).
JONCAS and PAVILANIS: Canad. med. Ass. J. 82, 1108 (1960).
WALKER et al.: Canad. med. Ass. J. 83, 1266 (1960).
McLEAN et al.: Canad. med. Ass. J. 85, 496 (1961).
RAMOS-ALVAREZ and OLARTE: Amer. J. Dis. Child. 107, 220 (1964).

1960) and children (BERGAMINI and BONETTI, 1960) occur with type 11. On the other hand several ECHO viruses have spread widely (e.g. ECHO 15, MOSCOVICI et al., 1959) in nurseries, without ill effect, or encountered more often among well than among sick children (e.g. type 19, CRAMBLETT et al., 1962). Other serotypes isolated from infants with gastroenteritis are summarized in Table 4.

The variable frequency of encountering ECHO viruses among infants and children with respect to time and place is illustrated in Table 5. RAMOS-ALVAREZ and SABIN (1958), and RAMOS-ALVAREZ and OLARTE (1964) have recovered enteroviruses more often in children with diarrhea than in nondiarrheal controls. In other studies, recovery rates between patient and control groups were essentially similar (YOW et al., 1963). In all studies, viruses recovered from children with diarrhea were of the same groups found in the control children, the only difference being that of frequency. Similar findings may relate to *Salmonella* and pathogenic *Escherichia* (RAMOS-ALVAREZ and OLARTE, 1964). Although pathogenic bacteria and viruses may be harbored by the same patient, the data do not signify correlation in terms of increased pathogenicity. Gastroenteritis may develop among the control patients; lack of close follow-up of these individuals may introduce a bias, as has been pointed out (RAMOS-ALVAREZ and OLARTE, 1964) in criticism of earlier observations. There are still other factors related to pathogenesis, namely implantation of the right seed in a fertile soil; undoubtedly these conditions vary within the universe. Considering data reviewed here there is little doubt that ECHO virus serotypes cause gastroenteritis, which is followed by specific antibody responses. Some strains disseminate widely, even to adults finding within the alimentary tract cells uniquely susceptible to injury, or capable of withstanding cytocidal effects during viral replication.

4. The Respiratory Tract

Pharyngitis and cervical lymphadenitis are common expressions during infection from various ECHO viruses. Mild febrile respiratory illnesses are associated with types 3, 6, and 20 (ROSEN et al., 1958; CRAMBLETT et al., 1958; SACHTLEBEN and MUNK, 1961; ROSEN et al., 1964). Types 1 and 6, in Japan (quoted by MATUMOTO, 1962) have similar associations; adults were involved in the type 6 outbreak. Photophobia and conjunctivitis occurred among these patients. Diarrhea may develop. A syndrome simulating influenza has been reported for type 7 (ALBANO and SALVAGGIO, 1960). ECHO 11 has been associated with acute upper respiratory tract infections of children (PHILIPSON and ROSEN, 1959), some of whom developed subglottic croup. Adults accidentally or voluntarily infected with types 11, 19, 20, and 25 (children, also, see REILLY et al., 1963) may develop fever, coryza, pharyngitis and cervical adenitis; occasionally, adults developed diarrhea also.

5. Other Organ Systems

Pericarditis and myocarditis have been associated only rarely with types 1, 3, 6, 9, and 19 ECHO viruses (JOHNSON et al., 1961; KAVELMAN et al., 1961; SELWYN et al., 1963; KIBRICK, 1964). Pleurodynia has been noted during infection with types 1 and 9 (SOLOMON et al., 1959; KANTOR and HSIUNG, 1962; KARZON et al., 1962). Mild, apparently transitory alterations of liver function have been reported for types 4 and 9 (MALHERBE et al., 1957; SOLOMON et al., 1959). Orchitis has been reported in association with ECHO 9 (SANFORD and SULKIN, 1959). The point should be made that a firm association of specific cause and effect in the involvement of these various organs has not been established. For additional observations the reader is referred to several reviews on the status of ECHO viruses in human disease (SANFORD and SULKIN, 1959; KIBRICK, 1964).

B. Pathogenesis

Sites of primary colonization and multiplication of ECHO viruses appear to be within cells localized in the alimentary tract. All 31 serotypes have been found in feces; many can be recovered from the oropharynx; most are not easily recovered from the nasopharynx. The cardinal features of infection indicate a variable but lingering period of virus multiplication at primary sites; viremia may intervene with translocation of virus to other organs. Infection may be clinically silent, or expressly manifest with injury of a number of accessory cellular targets.

1. Experimental Infections

a) Human Beings

Adult volunteers have been inoculated (intranasal/oropharyngeal) with ECHO viruses types 11, 20, and 25 (BUCKLAND et al., 1959, 1961; KASEL et al., 1965). Subjects who are free of specific antibodies often developed minor respiratory illnesses (nasal congestion, sore throat, cough, lymphadenitis, etc.), as a rule without significant fever. Each serotype was readily recovered from pharyngeal and fecal samples for periods ranging from several days to 3 weeks. In the case of ECHO 20, peak concentrations of virus ($TCID_{50}$/gm) were $\sim 10^{3.0}$ in the pharynx and $\sim 10^{4.5}$ in the feces. Specific antibodies developed among volunteers from whom these viruses were recovered.

b) Chimpanzees

Types 2, 3, 4, 6, and 9 given orally, or parenterally to chimpanzees failed to induce overt signs of infection (ITOH and MELNICK, 1957; YOSHIOKA and HORSTMANN, 1960). Nevertheless several serotypes were readily recovered from the pharynx and stools of animals; during the first week, mean concentrations of virus (type 6) found were in the pharynx $10^{2.7}$, and in feces $10^{3.7}$ $TCID_{50}$/gm. In orally infected chimpanzees, virus excretion in the pharynx corresponded with, or even exceeded, the duration of excretion in feces (type 4). Viremia was encountered only with type 9 (a single isolate on the 1st day after parenteral inoculation with type 4 virus may represent overflow in situ).

c) Monkeys

Injury of neurones may be found in monkeys (M. mulatta and M. cynomolgus) after intramuscular inoculation or direct implantation of ECHO virus serotypes in the CNS (HAMMON et al., 1959a; LOU and WENNER, 1962). Following intramuscular inoculation with prototype strains focal lesions may be found in the brain stem and spinal cord of monkeys inoculated with types 1, 2, 3, 4, 6, 7, 10, 16, 19, and 24 (KAMITSUKA et al., 1961; LOU and WENNER, 1962). Similar lesions developed in monkeys inoculated intravenously or intraspinally with recently isolated strains of types 2, 7, 9, 14, 16, and 18; however, they were seldom found after oral or intramuscular inoculations. Types 7, 14, and 16 strains were associated with specific neuromuscular dysfunction; such effects were not discernible for others. Viruses were recovered from the blood and CSF. Animals inoculated orally with type 14 had positive blood cultures on the 4th and 6th days post-inoculation. ARNOLD and ENDERS (1959) obtained similar clinical responses, but less extensive neural damage after intrathecal (basal cistern) and/or intraspinal inoculation with types 6 and 16 ECHO viruses. The severe paralytic disease associated with ECHO 9 (VERLINDE and WILTERDINK, 1958), has been traced to poliovirus type 2 (vide supra). Myocarditis and pericarditis occasionally encountered in monkeys during ECHO virus infections may be specific effects; however, further observations are needed for firm association.

d) Mice

The prototype (Hill) strain of ECHO 9, isolated in monkey kidney cells from healthy American children lacks the property of mouse pathogenicity (RAMOS-ALVAREZ and SABIN, 1954; Committee on the ECHO Viruses, 1955). This strain and many others of ECHO virus type 9, isolated from healthy or diseased individuals are consistently nonpathogenic for newborn mice and cannot multiply, or be absorbed by newborn mouse tissues, even with maximal doses and after passage in cell cultures. On the other hand there are many other isolates of this type, which either on primary isolation or after some preliminary passage in cell culture have shown marked paralytogenic activity in infant mice (GEAR, 1959; ARCHETTI et al., 1956; TYRRELL and SNELL, 1956; McLEAN and MEL-NICK, 1957; GODFREDSEN and VON MAGNUS, 1957; LAFOREST et al., 1957; BROHL et al., 1957; JOHNSON, 1957; EGGERS and SABIN, 1959). Several factors enhance the paralytogenic effect for newborn mice (ARCHETTI et al., 1959; EGGERS and SABIN, 1959). Various strains show heterogeneity in plaque morphology and in their rates of absorption onto monkey kidney cells. Rapidly absorbing viruses are likely to be pathogenic for mice. Other factors relating to mouse-pathogenicity include dose, selection of pathogenic variants, and variations in susceptibility of mice. Paralytogenic virus stocks may be obtained either by passage in susceptible tissue cultures, or by serial "blind" passage in mice. Since a large dose ($\sim 10^6 \pm 1.0$ TCID$_{50}$) is required for the paralytic response, serial passage in tissue culture and in mice appears to be primarily a titer-building function ($\sim 10^8 \pm 1.0$ PFU/gm); a secondary, but equally important function in mice is the selection of mouse-pathogenic variants as they arise. If the fraction of mouse-pathogenic particles comprising the total viral population is small they might be missed, since there is a race between mouse and virus. The mouse is relatively refractory to the paralytogenic effect after the 5th day of life. Therefore the rate of replication in the newborn mouse must be rapid enough to produce the minimal paralytogenic dose within the allotted time; otherwise, slow replication means no clinical effect and the mouse-pathogenic variants are lost. Mouse-pathogenic variants may be lost also by passage in monkey stable (MS) kidney cells (LI, 1959).

2. Natural Infection

ECHO viruses are readily recovered from the pharynx and lower alimentary tract of infected human beings. The data regarding the duration of excretion, and relative concentrations of virus in the oropharynx vary greatly; some observations indicate persistence for several weeks (see section on epidemiology). In general, however, larger concentrations of virus, shed over a longer period apply to fecal discharges. These measurements, however, could be quite erroneous considering differences in sampling procedures, potential concentration in the large intestine, and quantitative differences of susceptible cells in the general milieu. The prolonged excretion of virus in the pharynx of chimpanzees suggest that similar events may apply to human beings; very few data are available for the early phases of infection. Evidence supporting occult infection has been obtained for ECHO 9, wherein viremia may occur 6 days before onset of clinical illness. Viremia accompanies infection with types 4, 6, 9, 11, 14, 16, and 18. The single record of ECHO 6 in blood relates to a rapidly fatal paralytic illness in a 7-year-old girl who died 7 days after onset (MOORE et al., 1964). Virus was not recovered from oropharynx, stool or CNS tissues. Antibody neutralizing (1:8) type 6 virus was found in only 1 of 6 family associates. Other isolations are less disputable; they have been obtained from many children with minor illnesses, cutaneous eruptions, or aseptic meningitis. Excepting type 16, all serotypes noted above have been recovered from CSF. Additional serotypes found therein include types 1, 2, 5, 7, 12, 15, 19, 20, 23, 25, 30, and 31. ECHO virus type 11 has been recovered from cutaneous lesions.

ECHO viruses have been recovered from various organs after death. All reports relate to infants and children. Types 2 and 9 have been recovered from the CNS, type 9 from the lung of a neonate, and type 19 from the brain, lung, heart, liver, spleen, lymph node and intestine (but not from blood) of a premature infant (STEIGMAN, 1958; VERLINDE and WILTERDINK, 1958; BUTTER-FIELD et al., 1963; RAWLS et al., 1964). SELWYN et al. (1963) failed to recover type 3 virus from the CNS of a 12-year-old girl whose illness simulated bulbar poliomyelitis, although type 3 virus was recovered from the feces. Post mortem studies failed to demonstrate neuronal injury, but revealed pancarditis. Virus studies of extraneural tissues were not reported. In these studies the concentration of virus found in body fluids and tissues varied widely. Levels of viremia for ECHO 9 ranged from 8 to 174 $TCID_{50}$/ml; high concentrations ($10^{5.3}$ $TCID_{50}$) may be found in the pharynx, whereas titer values for feces range from $\sim 10^{1.0}$ to $10^{4.0}$ $TCID_{50}$/gm. Concentrations of ECHO 19 in tissues noted above ranged from $10^{1.8}$ to $10^{3.5}$ (unit volume not stated). The high concentration of ECHO 9 in CNS tissues ($10^{6.5}$ $TCID_{50}$/gm) was mentioned earlier.

Many facets in the pathogenesis of ECHO virus infections await definition. At the cellular level, those include a) cell type(s) supporting first cycles of virus multiplication, b) nature of injury to primary target cell(s), c) mode of transport to secondary and tertiary target cells, and d) alterations in homeostasis permissive of overt disease. Thus far in our knowledge it would appear that the course of events resembles very closely that of poliomyelitis, and, like the latter, there are still areas of ignorance. However, it seems reasonable that primary sites of colonization are in the alimentary tract, and that there is little translocation in the majority of patients. But there are notable exceptions depending in part at least on host susceptibility, the virus, and other poorly defined parameters which allow penetration leading to viremia and transport of virus to secondary and tertiary cell targets. Viremia precedes injury to tertiary targets (e.g. CNS) and terminates usually with the intervention of clinical disease, at a time when antibodies have already appeared. One of the major unknown features of pathogenesis relates to the nature of the secondary targets (e.g. reticulo-endothelial cells) wherein rapid growth of virus leads to an incremental upsurge of viremia, which in turn largely distinguishes whether infection will manifest itself as disease.

Table 6. *Sites of Recovery of ECHO Viruses in Human Beings*

Serotype	Source					
	Feces	Pharynx	CSF	Blood	Urine	Other tissues
1	+		+			
2	+		+			CNS
3	+	+				
4	+	+	+	+		
5	+		+			
6	+	+	+	+		
7	+	+	+			
8	+					
9	+	+	+	+	+	CNS, Lung, Skin
11	+	+	+	+		Skin
12	+		+			
13	+					
14	+	+	+	+	+	
15	+		+			
16	+	+	+	+		
17	+					
18	+	+	+	+		
19	+	+	+			CNS, Lung, Heart, Liver, etc.
20	+	+	+			
21	+					
22	+	+				
23	+		+			
24	+					
25	+	+	+			
26	+					
27	+					
29	+	+				
30	+		+			
31	+		+			
32	+					
33	+					

C. Immunity

Type-specific humoral antibodies develop during the infectious state. Neutralizing antibodies appear within a fortnight after alimentary infection (ROSEN
et al., 1958). They are found either at onset of meningitis, or shortly thereafter
(24 hours) with ECHO virus type 9 (SABIN et al., 1958). As noted in the section
on pathogenesis disease may only develop in later stages of infection. Neutralizing antibodies not only appear early, but persist for many months or years.
Usually, HI and CF antibodies are found a few days later. For ECHO 6, neutralizing and HI antibodies reach peak concentrations early in the second week after
onset. Neutralizing antibody persist without appreciable decline for at least
3 years. HI antibody decline rapidly during the ensuing weeks, but are still
detectable during the same period. On the other hand, the CF antibodies after
reaching peak level (10—24 days) fall rapidly, and if detectable are only barely
so at the end of 3 years (BUSSELL et al., 1962b). Somewhat different results
were obtained for ECHO 16; complement fixing antibodies fell moderately
within 1 to 2 years, and persisted thereafter for at least 3 to 6 years, as did neu-

tralizing antibodies (NEVA and MALONE, 1959 b). These findings apply to individuals with clinical disease; data relating to inapparent infection (HENIGST et al., 1961) indicate responses of similar magnitudes and durations.

Premature and full-term infants often receive antibodies from their mothers. CRAMBLETT et al. (1961) noted that infant and maternal titers were not equivalent for several ECHO viruses. Neutralizing antibodies for types 1, 2, 8, 11, and 20 were frequently less than the mother's titer. Clinical infection in newborn infants with pre-existing passively acquired antibodies has been noted (EICHEN-WALD and KOTSEVALOV, 1960) for type 9. Nevertheless the newborn infant, with but few exceptions for all the ECHO viruses, has not borne a major burden of clinical disease; infection rates may be high but disease incidence is relatively low. Manifestations of illness for most (but not all) ECHO viruses appear to be milder in premature and newborn infants than in older children. Inasmuch as the modulating factor could not be ascribed to passively-transferred antibodies, attenuation must be founded on other less specific host-virus reactions.

While antibodies, either passively or actively acquired, may sometimes prevent, and also modulate the clinical expression of disease, it is abundantly clear that they may not preclude infection. Examples can be cited where ECHO viruses were recovered from the pharynx and feces of sero-positive individuals. On the other hand, sero-negative individuals acquiring infection may not develop other traceable signs. Recovery from infection is related to a number of events, among which are quenching of initial rapid virus multiplication, elimination (or sequestration) of virus, and a coincidental state of clinical refractoriness leading to repair and immunity. While not much is known about nonspecific resistance, and those factors responsible for it in relation to ECHO viruses, much has been written for polio- and Coxsackie viruses. Those relate in the present context largely to temporal events of infection with several enteroviruses, and their capacities to interfere with the host's response to another. The implantation of attenuated polioviruses (vaccine strains) may be significantly reduced when administered during high prevalence of other enteroviruses. Conversely, a *temporary* obliteration of the usual enteric viral flora may occur following massive application of oral poliovirus vaccine; however, following cessation of poliovirus excretion other enteroviruses reappear (RAMOS-ALVAREZ et al., 1959; SABIN et al., 1960; DÖMOK et al., 1962). In monkeys there is suggestive evidence that ECHO 7 interferes with systemic invasion of poliovirus type 1 (KONO et al., 1963). While there is fragmentary evidence of serologic cross-relationship between members of the major subgroups of human enteroviruses, none of the data strikes a confident note that immunity to one conveys protection to another serotype.

In summary, it would appear that immunity to infection and disease with the ECHO viruses relates most cogently not only to the presence, but also to the concentration of specific humoral antibodies. On the other hand nonspecific environmental factors may exert an influence on endemic and epidemic prevalences — hence indirectly reducing risk of disease. Once the virus has reached secondary target organs, specific antibody appears to be of lesser importance than some other responses (e.g. release of interferon, inflammatory cellular reactions, etc.) in determining repair and recovery.

D. Epidemiology

ECHO viruses are obligatory human commensals whose survival depends on successful implantation in susceptible cells of the alimentary tract. Man is the only known natural host. There is as yet no singular study delineating with certainty the mode of spread. The situation is like that of poliomyelitis where virus may be recovered from the pharynx for about a week, and in feces for longer intervals (see below). The cumulative data for many ECHO viruses suggest a direct person-to-person oral transfer of human excrement. Such may be the main avenue; however, for some, notably type 9, other modes of transfer might have been operative. The extensive rapid waves of infection occurring throughout Europe in 1956, the simultaneous upsurge in separate geographic areas, and the very rapid recruitment of susceptibles resemble those observed for influenza rather than poliomyelitis. SABIN et al. (1958) estimated that 4400 persons in Milwaukee (pop. 365,000) acquired infection during a single week. Having in view also the high concentrations of ECHO 9 in the oropharynx, the possibility and indeed the probable person-to-person transfer of pharyngeal virus cannot be ignored. As yet there is no evidence of widespread outbreaks through common vehicles such as milk, water, or insect vectors.

1. Geographic Prevalence

ECHO viruses and antibodies thereto have been found in people throughout the world. A geographical mapping of isolates has been tabulated by GELFAND (1961). We can add only a few recent isolates principally from the Western Hemisphere, Europe and Great Britain. There is practically no information for type 21. Serum-neutralizing antibodies for types 6, 7, 8, 9, 11, and 14 indicate that they also prevail in Arctic North America, South America, Asia and Africa (KALTER, 1962). Knowledge on the intensity of infection in many parts of the world is still fragmentary.

2. Season and Climate

In temperate climates epidemics (we know of none in tropical areas) have occurred during the warm months. In our clinics even sporadic cases are rarely encountered during the winter (Eskimos may provide an exception). The striking seasonal distribution of ECHO 9 during the outbreak in Milwaukee is illustrated in Fig. 4.

Another parameter measuring the seasonal frequency of infection is graphically depicted in Fig. 4. Top panels illustrate the frequency (per cent) of encountering enteroviruses among infants and children. These data point up a major prevalence of enteroviruses during the warmest months. Infection rates were lowest during the winter and spring, rose rapidly to reach their maxima during the summer, and gradually declined during the autumn. GELFAND (1961) plotted the seasonal distribution of enterovirus subgroups and found ECHO virus frequencies to peak about a month after polio- and Coxsackie viruses. Whether the observation is meaningful is not known. As far as climate is concerned, studies from the southern USA, and the Belgian Congo strongly suggest

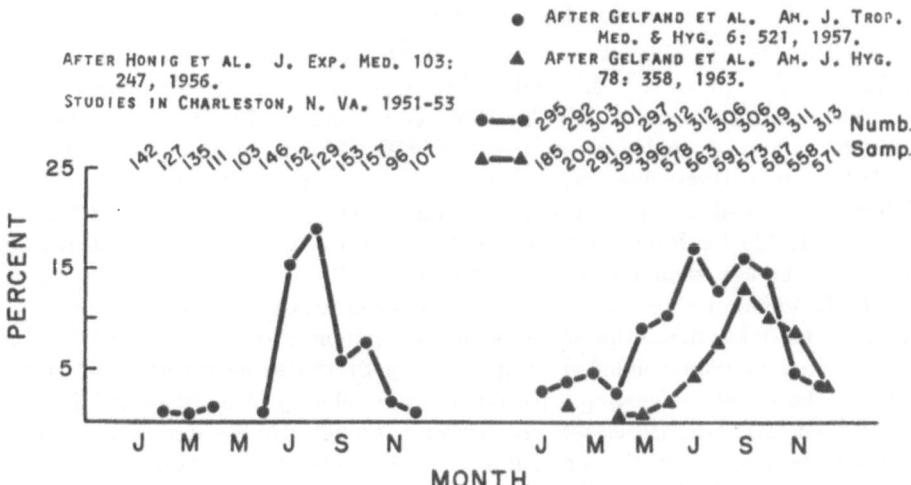

THE CHARLESTON STUDIES REPRESENT ALL ENTEROVIRUSES DETECTED IN FECES. THE LOUISIANA STUDIES (● SYMBOL) REPRESENT NON-POLIO ENTEROVIRUSES, AS DOES THE COMPOSITE CHART (▲ SYMBOL) FOR ENTEROVIRUSES ISOLATED FROM HEALTHY CHILDREN IN 6 CITIES (USA) 1960.

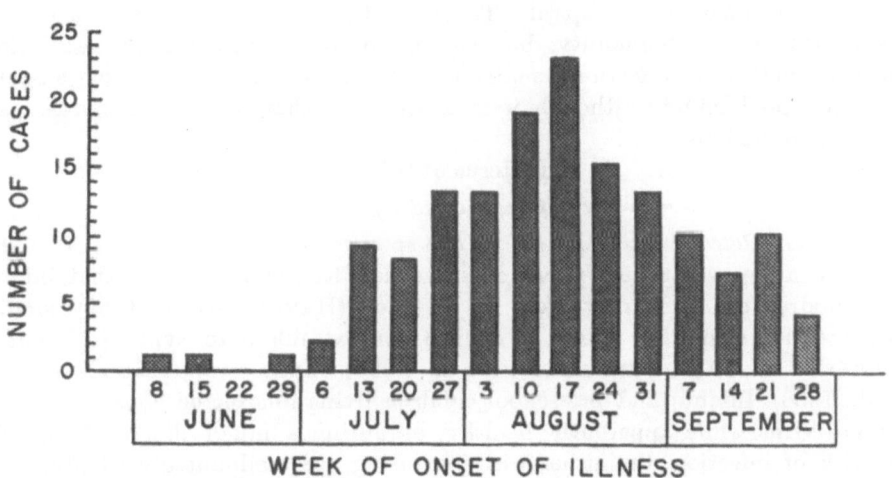

Fig. 4. Seasonal prevalence of enteroviruses in several population groups (top panel); a comparison of those with seasonal prevalence of illness from ECHO virus, type 9 (bottom panel). After SABIN et al., Amer. J. Dis. Child. 96, 197—219 (1958).

that infection rates have less seasonal fluctuation than in cooler latitudes. In tropical areas, however, ECHO viruses appear to be endemically prevalent throughout the year.

3. Secular Variations in Prevalence

Epidemicity. Epidemics caused by ECHO viruses are generally localized and sporadic in character; the epidemic serotype may differ from place to place, however, during the same year. In 1955, two different ECHO viruses were responsible for local epidemics in Iowa (ECHO 4) and Buffalo (ECHO 6) New York. In 1956, Coxsackie virus Group B, type 4 prevailed in Iowa, whereas ECHO 4 prevailed in Buffalo and in Melbourne. During the same period ECHO 9 was responsible for large epidemics in Western Europe, and in Great Britain; similar outbreaks soon occurred in Canada (1961) and in the United States (1957). Pandemic waves have not been recognized for other ECHO viruses. However, GELFAND has noted that the subclinical "epidemic" of infection with ECHO 7 in Louisiana in 1956 coincided with recovery of the same serotype in various parts of the world, suggesting a pandemic wave, chiefly of inapparent infections. In 1954, ECHO 6 was associated with aseptic meningitis in Sweden, Massachusetts and Rhode Island; in the preceding and subsequent year this serotype was encountered widely in the United States. In recent years similar observations pertain to ECHO 30 in Scotland, the United States and Canada. In 1959, two enteroviruses were accountable for CNS disease in Scotland (LANDSMAN et al., 1961; DUNCAN, 1961). During late spring and summer, Coxsackie virus A 7 prevailed, whereafter in the second half of the year, ECHO 30 (Frater) was the main cause of disease.

Endemicity. Enteroviruses are accountable also for sporadic illness, some of which are studied in hospitals. These are heralds undoubtedly of a greater prevalence in the community, but because of infrequent clinical association, the true evidence of infection remains uncertain. As a rule, in any year singular serotypes predominate although it is exceptional that other enteroviruses are not encountered also.

4. Patterns of Infection

a) Risks According to Age

Infection Rates. Data relating to age-specific infection rates are available for only a few serotypes. Those obtained for ECHO 7 indicate that infants and children are primary targets of infection (HENIGST et al., 1961); similar findings in a somewhat different clinical context relate to types 4, 6, and 9 (LEHAN et al., 1957; WINKELSTEIN et al., 1957; SABIN et al., 1958; KLEINMAN et al., 1958). Infants and pre-school children living in affected households often excrete virus while apparently healthy, or during a minor illness. As a rule, the risk of infection diminishes with increasing age, undoubtedly wholly, or at least in major part due to immunity engendered from antecedent infection.

Clinical Rates. Age-specific attack rates based on reported cases emphasize a preponderant risk of youth. During many outbreaks, rates of children exceed those of infants; rates in young adults often correspond with those of children. These rates relate largely to the risk of aseptic meningitis; in contrast, the highest incidence of rash with ECHO 9, 16 and others (e.g. types 2, 4, 18, etc.)

Table 7. *Age Distribution of Patients Presenting with Aseptic Meningitis*

Age groups (years)	ECHO virus											
	Type 4				Type 6			Type 9		Type 16	Type 30	
	Iowa USA	Buffalo USA	Scotland UK	Kentucky USA	Conn. USA	Buffalo USA	Belgium	Scotland UK	Milwaukee USA	Mass. USA	Scotland UK	Minn. USA
<1	54[1]	15	24	0	0	12	10	7	4	~83	1	2
1—4		43	~33	12	30	40	14	17	22		16	
5—9		28	~25	54	~60	25	23	50	30	~12	30	19
10—14		14	≤18		~10	23	15	26	19		29	21
Over 15	46			34			37		25	5	24	58
All ages	67	82	42	52	21	156	195	178	149	2346	67	58

[1] Expressed as per cent of total in each column. Many, but not all, patients were virus-positive.

References:

Type 4: LEHAN et al.: Amer. J. Hyg. **66**, 63 (1957). KARZON et al.: Amer. J. Dis. Child. **101**, 610 (1961). BELL: Lancet **1**, 1195 (1963). RAY et al.: Amer. J. Epidem. **84**, 253 (1966).

Type 6: DAVIS and MELNICK: Proc. Soc. exp. Biol. (N.Y.) **92**, 839, (1956). WINKELSTEIN et al.: Amer. J. publ. Hlth **47**, 741 (1957).

Type 9: NIHOUL et al.: Amer. J. Hyg. **66**, 102 (1957). LANDSMAN et al.: A Combined Scottish Study. Scot. med. J. **9**, 141 (1964). SABIN et al.: Amer. J. Dis. Child. **96**, 197 (1958).

Type 16: NEVA et al.: J. Amer. med. Ass. **155**, 544 (1954).

Type 30: LANDSMAN et al.: A Combined Scottish Study. Brit. med. J. **2**, 597 (1961). KLEINMAN et al.: J. Amer. med. Ass. **187**, 90 (1964).

has been during infancy and early childhood. These desiderata relate only to proportionalities, and it scarcely needs be pointed out that infants develop meningitis and adults cutaneous lesions.

b) Familial Aggregation

ECHO viruses spread rapidly within the microcosm of the family, particularly in those with young children. Children acquiring infection elsewhere introduce these viruses to susceptible members of their households. Secondary cases often occur within a few days of one another. Five of 7 familial associates observed during an ECHO 4 outbreak became ill within 14 days; onset of meningitis in 4 children occurred within a 4-day period (CHIN et al., 1957). Essentially similar relationships apply to 7 of 8 members of a family infected with ECHO 9 virus (FAULKNER et al., 1957), and to 8 members of several families introduced to ECHO 7 virus during a reunion (KLEINMAN et al., 1962). SABIN et al. (1958) recovered 58 ECHO 9 strains from 104 persons of 22 families in which one or more members had meningitis. Similar observations pertain to type 9 (ROTEM and LAUSANNE, 1957; NIHOUL et al., 1957; BAUMANN et al., 1957; GALPINE et al., 1958, and others), type 6 (WINKELSTEIN et al., 1957; JOHNSSON et al., 1957), type 16 (NEVA, 1956), and type 30 (DUNCAN, 1961; KLEINMAN et al., 1964). The spread of infection among children lodged in summer camps may be less inclusive than in families (PAFFENBARGER et al., 1959), possibly due to less intense and discontinuous exposure to an index case already well along in the infectious state.

c) Sex, Race and Socio-economic Status

Males develop overt disease more often than females. Since serological enquiry indicates similar infection rates in both sexes the basis for differences in disease incidence must relate to other parameters. Increased susceptibility or natural resistance among the human races has not been recognized. The course of infection, and possibly the risk of disease may depend on socio-economic factors, namely crowding, poor hygienic milieu, the level of "herd" immunity, among others. Numerous studies have emphasized, particularly during the early years of life, differing breadths of antigenic experiences, differing velocities of infection and variable risks of disease. These studies indicate not only a reciprocal relationship between social-deprivation and risk of infection, but also, among the more affluent, a somewhat greater risk of disease.

d) The Virus Carrier State

Feces. ECHO viruses are readily found in feces during the first week of infection. Excretion rates may fall (e.g. types 6, 9, 20, 25, etc.) sharply during the second week. Fox (1964) found the mean duration of excretion for types 2, 3, 6, 11, 18, 25, and 27 to be 14 days (range 1—28 days). HENIGST et al. (1961) established a mean interval of 24 days for ECHO 7. Young children (i.e. ≤ 5 years) are apt to shed virus in feces longest, but the rule is not inviolate, for with type 7 the longest observed periods of excretion (≤ 3.5 months) were among older children. Virus concentrations are highest early in infection; some median values expressed in $TCID_{50}/gm$ for feces were $10^{5.5}$ for type 7, $10^{4.5}$ for type 8 and $10^{3.0}$ for type 12

Table 8. *Virus Recovery Rates by Age among Index Patients and Their Familial Associates*

ECHO 6

Age (years)	Index cases No. examined	Index cases positive %	Family associates No. examined	Family associates positive %
0— 4	16	44	21	52
5— 9	53	68	17	41
10—14	29	66	11	9
15—19	12	67	4	0
20 and over	17	47	57[1]	17
Totals	127	61	110	26

ECHO 7

Age (years)	Family associates No. examined	Family associates positive %
<2	23	88
2	18	89
3— 4	27	67
5— 9	40	55
10—14	10	40
Totals	128	69

ECHO 9

Age (years)	Index cases No. examined	Index cases positive %	Family associates No. examined	Family associates positive %
0— 4	29	87	6	33
5—14	15	87	6	17
15 and over	13	77	23	13
Totals	57	84	32	31

ECHO 9

Age (years)	Cases No. examined	Cases positive %
0— 2	19	90
3— 5	11	91
6—10	7	57
10 and under	37	84
10 and over	19	44
Totals	56	70

ECHO 30

Age (years)	Cases[2] No. examined	Cases[2] positive %
0— 5	12	18
6—10	20	30
11—15	19	28
16—25	10	15
25 and over	6	9
Totals	67	100

[1] Includes 4 contacts of unknown age. [2] Only virus positive cases entered in Table.

References:

Type 6: WINKELSTEIN et al.: Amer. J. publ. Hlth 47, 741 (1957).
Type 7: HENIGST et al.: Amer. J. trop. Med. Hyg. 10, 759 (1961).
Type 9: SABIN et al.: Amer. J. Dis. Child. 96, 197 (1958).
Type 9: LEPOW et al.: Pediatrics 26, 12 (1960).
Type 30: LANDSMAN et al.: A Combined Scottish Study, Brit. med. J. 2, 597 (1961).

ECHO viruses. Data essentially similar to type 7 have been obtained for types 3, 9, and 20 (SABIN et al., 1958, WIGAND and SABIN, 1962; ROSEN et al., 1958, 1964).

Pharynx. ECHO viruses may be recovered from the oropharynx during infection. ECHO 9 virus was found in the oropharynx of a familial contact two days prior to onset of illness. Among 8 patients varying concentrations of ECHO 9 virus (10 to 125,000 $TCID_{50}$/swab) were encountered during the first week of illness. The virus recovery rate (35 patients) was 75% during the first, and dropped to 10% during the second week (WIGAND and SABIN, 1962). On the other hand, FOX (1964) was able to detect pharyngeal virus in only less than half of the

Table 9. *Approximate Duration of Virus Carrier State: Frequency Distribution in Weeks, Based on Time of Initial Virus Isolation or Onset of Meningitis*

ECHO virus serotype	For feces								For pharynx							
	Week								Week							
	1		2		3		4		1		2		3		4	
	No.	%	No.	%	No.	%	No.	%	No.	%	No.	%	No.	%	No.	%
3	16	69	10	60	7	43	6	33	10	30	10	30	—	—	—	—
6	88	~25	88	~8	88	≤3	—	—	—	—	+[1]	—	—	—	—	—
7	—	—	96	45	—	—	96	26	—	—	—	—	—	—	—	—
9	—	86[2]	—	74[2]	—	37[2]	—	37[2]	—	—	—	—	—	—	—	—
9	101	57	45	27	—	—	17	16	17	35	3	0	—	—	—	—
20	84	70	69	42	54	28	58	21	6	17	6	34	1	0	1	0
25	15	40	14	0	14	7	14	7	—	—	—	—	—	—	—	—
29	3	100	2	67	—	—	—	—	3	0	—	—	—	—	—	—

Adapted from the following references:

Type 3   ROSEN et al.: Amer. J. Hyg. **79**, 163 (1964).
Type 6   KARZON and BARRON: Pediatrics **29**, 409 (1962).
Type 7   HENIGST et al.: Amer. J. trop. Med. Hyg. **10**, 759 (1961).
Type 9   SABIN et al.: Amer. J. Dis. Child. **96**, 187 (1958).
Type 9   NIHOUL et al.: Amer. J. Hyg. **66**, 102 (1957).
Type 20   ROSEN et al.: Amer. J. Hyg. **67**, 300 (1958); CRAMBLETT et al.: Pediatrics **21**, 168 (1958).
Type 25   ROSEN et al.: Amer. J. Hyg. **79**, 1 (1964).
Type 29   ROSEN et al.: Amer. J. Hyg. **79**, 7 (1964).

[1] From data mentioned in text; [2] Total number tested = 152, but number tested for each interval is not given. No. = number tested, % = per cent positive tests.

individuals infected with types 2, 3, 6, 11, 18, 25, and 27, and usually only on a single occasion, thereby estimating a mean carrier state of 1 day! These data are dissimilar to those obtained by ROSEN et al. (1958, 1964) for type 3, as well as for types 20 and 25, wherein it is shown that these viruses may persist in a third of the subjects for at least two weeks.

ECHO 9 virus was not recovered from the anterior nasopharynx, and only once (8 patients) was it recovered from the anterior portion of the mouth (SABIN et al., 1958).

5. Extra-human Reservoirs

Fecal soilage leaves its imprint in nature. When human excretion rates are highest, ECHO and other enteric viruses, and bacteria may be found in raw sewage where their presence provides an index of prevealing human flora. Enteroviruses may not be inactivated by primary and secondary sedimentation, or by usual procedures of chlorination of water (vide supra; also MELNICK et al., 1954; KELLY, 1957; KELLY and SANDERSON, 1961; OZERES et al., 1961; LAPIN-LEIMU and PENTTINEN, 1963; LAMB et al., 1964). Thus effluents discharged into waterways may contribute to pollution for as far as a mile from the outfall.

Despite the wide distribution of these viruses in nature there are no indisputable instances of dissemination of virus to human beings by contaminated water, milk or milk products, or other edibles (e.g. shellfish, etc.). ECHO viruses types 1, 5, and 11 (RIORDAN et al., 1961) have been recovered from wild flies; under singular circumstances direct transmission to human beings very likely takes place from time to time. Despite the development of viremia, lasting several days, we know of no searches for ECHO viruses among blood-sucking arthropods.

Antibodies neutralizing types 6, 7, 8, and 9 have been found in sera of dogs (GELFAND, 1961). ECHO 6 viruses have been recovered from kennel dogs (PINDAK and CLAPPER, 1964); dogs inoculated with virus remained essentially healthy (PINDAK and CLAPPER, 1965). The type 8, or related virus recovered from swine has not been fully characterized (MOSCOVICI, C. personal communication). Picornaviruses of non-primate species have not been related either serologically or clinically to the human serotypes (PLUMMER, 1965).

VIII. Addendum

The literature review for this chapter was completed in November, 1965. A number of significant studies have since appeared; many recent studies are briefly mentioned below, following the format used in the text.

There is a current foment, and desired effort to reclassify viruses based on emerging physical and chemical properties (LWOFF and TOURNIER, 1966; MELNICK and McCOMBS, 1966).

The human kidney cell culture approaches the ideal for recovery of enteroviruses (and adenoviruses, as well) from rectal swabs (LEE et al., 1965). Human kidney cells and WI-38 cells were considered choice tissue cultures for most studies of enteric viruses. WALLIS et al. (1965) have described another rapid method for titration and typing of enteroviruses, and for measuring the neutralizing antibody response. The method utilizes tube cultures in which cell monolayers are grown on the bottom, and then overlaid with agar after virus or virus-serum inoculation. Fewer cells are needed for "seeding", and usually results are available in 1 to 3 days with rapidly growing viruses.

Plaque production of ECHO viruses is enhanced by $MgCl_2$ (25 mM), L-cysteine (1 mM) and pancreatin (WALLIS et al., 1966). Incorporation of DEAE-dextran in agar not only enhances, but also facilitates (larger) plaque development. (ROUHANDEH et al., 1966; FEORINO and HANNON, 1966).

Further studies have been reported on the chemical inhibition of enterovirus multiplication and the production of CPE in cell cultures. Using drug-sensitive and drug-dependent strains of poliovirus and ECHO virus type 12, guanidine and HBB are capable of interrupting ongoing viral RNA synthesis and virus production in single cells during the incremental phase of virus growth. These results indicate that enterovirus RNA polymerase (whose formation is inhibited by HBB and guanidine) is continuously synthesized during the exponential phase of viral replication (CALIGUIRI et al., 1965). In another study HBB markedly delayed (~35 hours) the appearance of CPE in monkey kidney cells infected with ECHO virus type 12. Although HBB inhibits virus reproduction, those cells initially infected with virus eventually degenerated. Emergence of HBB-resistant virus particles led to rapid spread of cellular infection and complete CPE (BABLANIAN et al., 1966).

Purified virions of several ECHO viruses have similar buoyant densities, slight variation in size and similar sedimentation rates (JAMISON and MAYOR, 1966; SCHAFFER and FROMMHAGEN, 1965). Density gradient centrifugation may be utilized for separation of virions, but not hemagglutinins of viruses possessing different buoyant densities (ENGLER and FOUAD, 1967).

The hemagglutinins of ECHO and other enteroviruses are under continuous scrutiny. This non-enzymatic union (with human 0 erythrocytes) is inhibited by specific sugars. Several ECHO viruses, when digested with β-glucosidase lost the HA property, suggesting the capsids may contain glycoproteins (LERNER et al., 1966a). There is evidence that a carbohydrate component is attached to the protein of the capsid. Aldoses inhibit the HA reaction. Enterovirus hemagglutination very likely involves the binding of a carbonyl group of an oligosaccharide side chain on the virus capsid to a specific receptor on the erythrocyte surface (LERNER et al., 1966b).

Hemagglutinins and viral infectivity have identical rates of thermal inactivation. Hemagglutinins are stabilized against thermal inactivation by mono- and bivalent cations, but this stabilization is dependent upon temperature, pH, and concentration of cation (PODOPLEKIN and IVANOVA, 1966). On the other hand, stabilization by certain organic compounds (cysteine, glutathione, etc.) were sometimes independent of pH, and temperature (PODOPLEKIN and NOVYSH, 1966). Patterns of stabilization with organic compounds were related in part to the antigenic characteristics of the virus, and the steric configuration of the compound. Blockade of sulfhydryl groups interfered with the stabilizing effect (PODOPLEKIN et al., 1966).

Several recent studies reemphasize the intratypic heterogeneity of the ECHO viruses. Serologic differences between the prototypic and Shropshire-like strains of type 4 have been found by double diffusion gel precipitin procedures (CONANT et al., 1966). Many freshly isolated strains of type 11 appear to be drifting away from the antigenic pattern of the prototype (SCHMIDT et al., 1966). In contrast type 19 strains possess serologic homogeneity but are heterogeneous with respect to kinds of plaques and hemagglutination patterns (DÖMÖK and SIMON, 1966).

Horses are choice animals for obtaining type-specific antisera for many of the enteroviruses (MELNICK and HAMPIL, 1965). Immunization of animals with viruses treated with molar MgCl$_2$ and concentrated (10×) by the MgAl carbonate method (HAMPIL et al., 1965) yielded high-titer type-specific antisera.

Several new clinical expressions have been introduced and several older ones reinforced. Types 21 and 22, and some additional unrelated viruses have been found in feces of infants dying unexpectedly (BALDUZZI and GREENDYKE, 1966); the association is uncertain. A similar situation applies to type 9 and glomerulonephritis (YUCEOGLU et al., 1966). On the other hand, two clinical features have received reinforcement. First, herpangina, in the past associated with Coxsackie viruses has been noted during infection with ECHO viruses types 9, 16 and 17 (CHERRY and JAHN, 1965). Second, there are additive reports on intervening neuromuscular disease, particularly for type 4 (KOPEL et al., 1965; MAJIMA et al., 1965), and type 9 (WILTERDINK et al., 1965).

Data reinforcing epidemiological data, entered in the text, relate largely to reports on additional outbreaks associated with type 4 (BOBROWSKI and TAYTACH, 1963; KON et al., 1965; KAWANA et al., 1965; and HINUMA et al., 1966), and type 6 (KAWANA, 1965). Several studies (PARKS et al., 1966; BEH-BEHANI and WENNER, 1966; BEHBEHANI, 1967) have noted the early appearance of ECHO viruses in the alimentary tract of infants and children with or without diarrhea. In Karachi types 1, 11, 14 and 19 were dominant types. In Teheran, types 11, 21 and 30 prevailed.

Continuing surveillance of enteroviruses in the U.S.A. (FROESCHLE et al., 1966) and in the United Kingdom (GAILBRAITH, 1965) have added a few new dimensions. The American studies indicate increased pathogenicity at several age levels. Children under one year of age are at greatest risk of CNS disease; the risk then diminishes up to 6 years, and then increases with increasing age. Longitudinal studies (FOX et al., 1966; SPIGLAND et al., 1966 and ELVEBACK et al., 1966) in New York City supplement data presented earlier in the Chapter on duration of excretion. ECHO viruses accounted for the smallest proportion of infections, and one of the shortest durations of virus shedding ($\sim$14 days). In terms of pathogenicity the enteroviruses recovered were only infrequently associated with frank neurologic disease; in general significant association was not established between infections and disease. Possibly related illnesses varied from 43% for adeno- and enteroviruses to 71% for rhinoviruses. The last series of papers contain comprehensive data and cannot be summarized in a brief statement.

In addition to ECHO 9, two type 6 strains are reported (VASILENKO and ATSEV, 1965) to produce paralysis and death in both suckling and young adult mice; the histological aspects were almost if not identical with those occurring in Coxsackie virus Group B infections. Type 6 was administered orally to dogs (beagles); they develop mild diarrhea, sometimes bloody; the virus was recovered in feces as long as 35 days after the initial feeding, and once, on the second post-inoculation day, in the blood (PINDAK and CLAPPER, 1966).

Finally, several interesting studies relate to methods used for recovery of enteroviruses from sewage and water. BERG et al. (1966) recovered viruses from drinking water by inoculating large volumes (isotonic) on cell cultures using sufficient number of cultures for precise quantitation. LUND and HEDSTRÖM (1966) used Albertson's two-phase system of aqueous polymers for recovery of virus from sewage. Enteroviruses may be detected in sewage without knowledge of existing illness, or before the appearance of clinical cases in the community (LUND et al., 1966).

Acknowledgments

The authors express their thanks to the several authors and publishers of journals for permission to reproduce the Figures entered in the text. Authors are cited. Acknowledgement is given Academic Press, Inc., New York, and The Rockefeller University Press, New York, for Figs. 2 and 3.

References

ALBANO, A., e L. SALVAGGIO: Sindrome similinfluenzale de virus ECHO tipo 7. Boll. Ist. sieroter. milan. **39,** 9 (1960).

ARCHETTI, I., G. R. DUBES, and H. A. WENNER: A comparative study of the prototypic Hill strain of ECHO virus, type 9, and several Coxsackie-like viruses related to it antigenically. Arch. ges. Virusforsch. **9,** 73 (1959).

ARCHETTI, I., A. FELICI, F. RUSSI, and C. FUA: Researches on the etiologic agent of the Marche meningoneuraxitis during the epidemic outbreak of the summer and autumn of 1955. Sci. med. ital. **5,** 321 (1956).

ARCHETTI, I., J. WESTON, and H. A. WENNER: Adaptation of ECHO viruses in HeLa cells; their use in complement fixation. Proc. Soc. exp. Biol. (N.Y.) **95,** 265 (1957).

ARNOLD, J. H., and J. F. ENDERS: Disease in Macacus monkeys inoculated with ECHO viruses. Proc. Soc. exp. Biol. (N.Y.) **101,** 513 (1959).

BABLANIAN, R., H. J. EGGERS, and I. TAMM: Inhibition of enterovirus cytopathic effects by 2-(α-hydroxybenzyl)-benzimidazole. J. Bact. **91,** 1289 (1966).

BALDUZZI, P. C., and R. M. GREENDYKE: Sudden unexpected death in infancy and viral infection. Pediatrics **38,** 201 (1966).

BALTIMORE, D., Y. BECKER, and J. E. DARNELL: Virus-specific double-stranded RNA in poliovirus-infected cells. Science **143,** 1034 (1964).

BALTIMORE, D., H. J. EGGERS, R. M. FRANKLIN, and I. TAMM: Poliovirus-induced RNA polymerase and the effect of virus-specific inhibitors on its production. Proc. nat. Acad. Sci. (Wash.) **49,** 843 (1963).

BARRON, A. L., and D. T. KARZON: Effect of pH on cytopathogenicity of orphan viruses. Proc. Soc. exp. Biol. (N.Y.) **94,** 393 (1957).

BARRON, A. L., and D. T. KARZON: Cultivation of enteroviruses in hamster kidney tissue culture. Proc. Soc. exp. Biol. (N.Y.) **100,** 316 (1959).

BARRON, A. L., and D. T. KARZON: Characteristics of ECHO 4 (Shropshire) virus isolated during epidemic of aseptic meningitis. J. Immunol. **87,** 608 (1961).

BARRON, A. L., and D. T. KARZON: Demonstration of ECHO 6 plaque variant. Bact. Proc. p. 134 (1962).

BARRON, A. L., and D. T. KARZON: Studies of mutants of ECHO-virus 6. I. Biologic and serologic characteristics. Amer. J. Epidem. **81,** 323 (1965).

BARSKI, G.: The significance of *in vitro* cellular lesions for classification of enteroviruses. Virology **18,** 152 (1962).

BARTELL, P., W. PIERZCHALA, and H. TINT: The adsorption of enteroviruses by activated attapulgite. J. Amer. pharm. Ass., sci. Ed. **49,** 1 (1960).

BAUMANN, T., M. BARBEN, R. MARTI, A. HASSLER und U. KRECH: Erkrankungen durch ECHO-Virus Typ 9. Eine epidemiologische, klinische und virologisch-serologische Studie. Schweiz. med. Wschr. **87,** 307 (1957).

BEHBEHANI, A. M.: Diarrhea in infants. J. Kans. med. Soc. **68,** 106 (1967).

BEHBEHANI, A. M., J. L. MELNICK, and M. E. DeBAKEY: Continuous cell strains derived from human atheromatous lesions and their viral susceptibility. Proc. Soc. exp. Biol. (N.Y.) **118,** 759 (1965).

BEHBEHANI, A. M., and H. A. WENNER: Antigenic relationship between strains of ECHO-virus types 6 and 30. Proc. Soc. exp. Biol. (N.Y.) **119,** 1158 (1965).

BEHBEHANI, A. M., and H. A. WENNER: Infantile diarrhea. A study of the etiologic role of viruses. Amer. J. Dis. Child. **111,** 623 (1966).

BELL, T. M., N. S. CLARK, and W. CHAMBERS: Outbreak of illness associated with ECHO type 7 virus. Brit. med. J. **2,** 292 (1963).

BENGTSSON, S.: Mechanism of dextran sulfate inhibition of attenuated poliovirus. Proc. Soc. exp. Biol. (N.Y.) **118,** 47 (1965).

BENYESH, M., E. C. POLLARD, E. M. OPTON, F. L. BLACK, W. D. BELLAMY, and J. L. MELNICK: Size and structure of ECHO, poliomyelitis, and measles viruses determined by ionizing radiation and ultrafiltration. Virology **5,** 256 (1958).

BERG, G., D. BERMAN, S. L. CHANG, and N. A. CLARKE: A sensitive quantitative method for detecting small quantities of virus in large volumes of water. Amer. J. Epidem. **83,** 196 (1966).

BERG, G., S. L. CHANG, and E. K. HARRIS: Devitalization of microorganisms by iodine. I. Dynamics of the devitalization of enteroviruses by elemental iodine. Virology **22,** 469 (1964).

BERG, G., N. C. CLARKE, and P. W. KABLER: Interrelationships among ECHO viruses types 1, 8, and 12. J. Bact. **83,** 556 (1962).

BERGAMINI, F., e F. BONETTI: Episodo epidemico di gastroenterite acuta da virus ECHO-11 in un Brefolrofio. Boll. Ist. sieroter. milan. **39,** 11 (1960).

BERGLUND, A., M. BÖTTIGER, T. JOHNSSON, and S. E. WESTERMARK: An outbreak of aseptic meningitis with a rubella-like rash caused by ECHO virus type 9. Arch. ges. Virusforsch. **8,** 294 (1958).

BERNKOPF, H., and A. ROSIN: Cytopathologic changes in tissue cultures of human amnionic cells infected with poliomyelitis, Coxsackie and ECHO viruses. Amer. J. Path. **33,** 1215 (1957).

BOBROWSKI, H., and F. Z. TAYTACH: The epidemic of lymphocytic meningitis caused by ECHO virus type 4. Przegl. epidem. (Warsaw) **17,** 301 (1963).

BROHL, I., K. HELMSTAEDT, H. LENNARTZ und G. MAASS: Über eine Epidemie von Coxsackie-Meningitis. Z. ärztl. Fortbild. **51,** 499 (1957).

BUCKLAND, F. E., M. L. BYNOE, L. PHILIPSON, and D. A. J. TYRRELL: Experimental infection of human volunteers with the U virus: a strain of ECHO virus type 11. J. Hyg. (Lond.) **57,** 274 (1959).

BUCKLAND, F. E., M. L. BYNOE, L. ROSEN, and D. A. J. TYRRELL: Inoculation of human volunteers with ECHO virus type 20. Brit. med. J. **1,** 397 (1961).

BUCKLAND, F. E., and D. A. J. TYRRELL: Loss of infectivity on drying various viruses. Nature (Lond.) **195,** 1063 (1962).

BUCKLEY, S. M.: Visualization of poliomyelitis virus by fluorescent antibody. Arch. ges. Virusforsch. **6,** 388 (1956).

BUCKLEY, S. M.: Cytopathology of poliomyelitis virus in tissue cultures. Fluorescent antibody and tinctorial studies. Amer. J. Path. **33,** 691 (1957).

BUSER, M., U. KRECH und S. MOESCHLIN: Zur Klinik und Verbreitung des Orphan-Virus (ECHO-Virus). Bericht über einen Fall mit paralytischer Myelitis durch ECHO-Virus Typ 4. Helv. med. Acta **24,** 434 (1957).

BUSSELL, R. H., D. T. KARZON, A. L. BARRON, and T. HALL: Hemagglutination-inhibiting, complement-fixing and neutralizing antibody responses in ECHO 6 infection, including studies on heterotypic responses. J. Immunol. 88, 47 (1962b).

BUSSELL, R. H., D. T. KARZON, and F. T. HALL: Hemagglutination and hemagglutination-inhibition studies with ECHO viruses. J. Immunol. 88, 38 (1962a).

BUTTERFIELD, J., C. MOSCOVICI, C. BERRY, and C. H. KEMPE: Cystic emphysema in premature infants. A report of an outbreak with the isolation of type 19 ECHO virus in one case. New Engl. J. Med. **268,** 18 (1963).

CALIGUIRI, L. A., H. J. EGGERS, N. IKEGAMI, and I. TAMM: A single-cell study of chemical inhibition of enterovirus multiplication. Virology **27,** 551 (1965).

CHEEVER, F. S.: Labeling techniques in diagnosis of enterovirus infection. Bact. Rev. **28,** 400 (1964).

CHERRY, J. D., and C. L. JAHN: Herpangina: The etiologic spectrum. Pediatrics **36,** 632 (1965).

CHERRY, J. D., A. M. LERNER, J. O. KLEIN, and M. FINLAND: ECHO 11 virus infections associated with exanthems. Pediatrics **32,** 509 (1963).

CHIN, T. D. Y., G. W. BERAN, and H. A. WENNER: An epidemic illness associated with a recently recognized enteric virus (ECHO virus type 4). II. Recognition and identification of the etiologic agent. Amer. J. Hyg. **66,** 76 (1957).

CHOPPIN, P. W., and H. J. EGGERS: Heterogeneity of Coxsackie B4 virus: Two kinds of particles which differ in antibody sensitivity, growth rate and plaque size. Virology **18,** 470 (1962).

CHOPPIN, P. W., and L. PHILIPSON: The inactivation of enterovirus infectivity by the sulfhydryl reagent p-chloromercuribenzoate. J. exp. Med. **113,** 713 (1961).

CLARKE, A., and J. P. STOTT: ECHO type 20. Letter to the editor. Brit. med. J. **1,** 900 (1961).

Committee on the ECHO Viruses: Enteric cytopathogenic human orphan (ECHO) viruses. Science 122, 1187 (1955).

Committee on Enteroviruses: National Foundation for Infantile Paralysis: The enteroviruses. Amer. J. publ. Hlth 47, 1556 (1957).

Committee on Human Picornaviruses: Picornaviruses: Classification of nine new types. Science 141, 153 (1963).

CONANT, R. M., A. M. BARRON, and F. MILGROM: Gel precipitation with ECHO 4 and other enteroviruses. Proc. Soc. exp. Biol. (N. Y.) 121, 307 (1966).

CRAMBLETT, H. G., L. ROSEN, R. H. PARROTT, J. A. BELL, R. J. HUEBNER, and N. B. McCULLOUGH: Respiratory illness in six infants infected with a newly recognized ECHO virus. Pediatrics 21, 168 (1958).

CRAMBLETT, H. G., F. D. WILKEN, M. LANGMACK, and J. PORTER: Patterns of transplacental transfer of neutralizing antibodies against ECHO virus types 1, 2, 8, 11, and 20. Amer. J. Hyg. 73, 90 (1961).

CRAMBLETT, H. G., H. L. MOFFETT, G. K. MIDDLETON, Jr., J. P. BLACK, H. SCHULEN-BERGER, and A. YONGUE: ECHO 19 virus infections. Clinical and laboratory studies. Arch. intern. Med. 110, 574 (1962).

CRANDELL, R. A., Y. P. HERMAN, J. R. GANAWAY, and W. H. NIEMANN: Susceptibility of primary cultures of feline renal cells to selected viruses. Proc. Soc. exp. Biol. (N.Y.) 106, 542 (1961).

CRAWFORD, M., A. D. MacCRAE, and J. N. O'REILLY: An unusual illness in young children associated with enteric virus. Arch. Dis. Childh. 31, 182 (1956).

DARDANONI, L., e P. ZAFFIRO: Sul potere emoagglutinanti di virus appartenente al gruppo ECHO. Boll. Ist. sieroter. milan. 37, 346 (1958).

DARDANONI, L., e P. ZAFFIRO: Identificazione di virus ECHO a mezzo della reazione di emoagglutino-inhibizione. Boll. Ist. sieroter. milan. 38, 441 (1959).

DARNELL, J. E., Jr., and T. K. SAWYER: The basis for variation in susceptibility to poliovirus in HeLa cells. Virology 11, 665 (1960).

DÖMÖK, I., E. MOLNÁR, A. JANCSÓ, and M. DÁNIEL: Enterovirus survey in children after mass vaccination with live attenuated polioviruses. Brit. med. J. 1, 743 (1962).

DÖMÖK, I., and M. SIMON: Intratypic variability of ECHO virus type 19. Virology 29, 553 (1966).

DUFFY, P. E., A. BELL, and M. G. MENEFEE: Morphology of ECHO 4 virus grown in monkey kidney tissue culture. Virology 16, 350 (1962).

DUNCAN, I. B. R.: Human thyroid tissue culture in diagnostic virology. Arch. ges. Virusforsch. 10, 490 (1960).

DUNCAN, I. B. R.: An outbreak of aseptic meningitis associated with a previously unrecognized virus. J. Hyg. (Lond.) 59, 181 (1961).

DUNCAN, I. B. R., and M. C. TIMBURY: Physical characteristics of Frater virus. Arch. ges. Virusforsch. 11, 365 (1961).

EGGERS, H. J., E. REICH, and I. TAMM: The drug-requiring phase in the growth of drug-dependent enteroviruses. Proc. nat. Acad. Sci. (Wash.) 50, 183 (1963).

EGGERS, H. J., and A. B. SABIN: Factors determining pathogenicity of variants of ECHO 9 virus for newborn mice. J. exp. Med. 110, 951 (1959).

EGGERS, H. J., and I. TAMM: Spectrum and characteristics of the virus inhibitory of 2-(α-hydroxybenzyl)-benzimidazole. J. exp. Med. 113, 657 (1961).

EGGERS, H. J., and I. TAMM: Synergistic effect of 2-(α-hydroxybenzyl)-benzimidazole and guanidine on picornavirus reproduction. Nature (Lond.) 199, 513 (1963a).

EGGERS, H. J., and I. TAMM: Drug dependence of enteroviruses: variants of Coxsackie A9 and ECHO 13 viruses that require 2-(α-hydroxybenzyl)-benzimidazole for growth. Virology 20, 62 (1963b).

EICHENWALD, H. F., A. ABABIO, A. M. ARKY, and A. P. HARTMAN: Epidemic diarrhea in premature and older infants caused by ECHO virus type 18. J. Amer. med. Ass. 166, 1563 (1958).

EICHENWALD, H. F., and O. KOTSEVALOV: Immunologic responses of premature and full-term infants to infection with certain viruses. Pediatrics 25, 829 (1960).

ELVEBACK, L. R., J. P. FOX, A. KETLER, C. D. BRANDT, F. E. WASSERMANN, and C. E. HALL: The virus watch program: A continuing surveillance of viral infections in metropolitan New York families. III. Preliminary report on association of infections with disease. Amer. J. Epidem. 83, 436 (1966).

ENDERS, J. F., T. H. WELLER, and F. C. ROBBINS: Cultivation of the Lansing strain of poliomyelitis virus in cultures of various human embryonic tissues. Science 109, 85 (1949).

ENGLER, R., and M. T. A. FOUAD: Differentiation of reoviruses and picornaviruses by density gradient centrifugation. Arch. ges. Virusforsch. 20, 29 (1967).

FABIYI, A., R. ENGLER, and D. C. MARTIN: Physical properties of infectious unit, hemagglutinin and complement-fixing antigen of ECHO virus 19. Arch. ges. Virusforsch. 14, 621 (1964).

FABIYI, A., and H. A. WENNER: Relationships between infectious virus, hemagglutinin and complement-fixing antigen of ECHO virus, type 19. Proc. Soc. exp. Biol. (N.Y.) 113, 81 (1963).

FAULKNER, R. S., A. J. MACLEOD, and C. E. VAN ROOYEN: Virus meningitis — seven cases in one family. Canad. med. Ass. J. 77, 439 (1957).

FELDMAN, H. A., and S. S. WANG: Sensitivity of various viruses to chloroform. Proc. Soc. exp. Biol. (N.Y.) 106, 736 (1961).

FEORINO, P. M., and W. H. HANNON: Use of DEAE dextran in agar overlays to enhance size of ECHO virus plaques. Publ. Hlth Rep. (Wash.) 81, 1015 (1966).

FOLEY, J. F., T. D. Y. CHIN, and C. R. GRAVELLE: Paralytic disease due to infection with ECHO virus type 9. New Engl. J. Med. 260, 924 (1959).

FORBES, J. A.: Meningitis in Melbourne due to ECHO virus. Part I. Clinical aspects. Med. J. Aust. 1, 246 (1958).

FOX, J. P.: Epidemiological aspects of coxsackie and ECHO virus infections in tropical areas. Amer. J. publ. Hlth 54, 1134 (1964).

FOX, J. P., L. R. ELVEBACK, I. SPIGAND, T. E. FROTHINGHAM, D. A. STEVENS, and M. HUGER: The Virus Watch Program: A continuing surveillance of viral infections in Metropolitan New York families. I. Overall plan, methods of collecting and handling information and a summary report of specimens collected and illnesses observed. Amer. J. Epidem. 83, 389 (1966).

FRANCIS, T., Jr., et al.: Evaluation of the 1954 Field Trial of Poliomyelitis Vaccine (Final Report) Michigan University Poliomyelitis Vaccine Evaluation Center, April 1957. Edwards Brothers, Inc., Ann Arbor, Michigan.

FROESCHLE, J. E., P. M. FEORINO, and H. M. GELFAND: A continuing surveillance of enterovirus infection in healthy children in six United States cities. II. Surveillance enterovirus isolates from cases of acute central nervous system disease. Amer. J. Epidem. 83, 455 (1966).

FROTHINGHAM, T. E.: ECHO virus type 9 associated with three cases simulating meningococcemia. New Engl. J. Med. 259, 484 (1958).

FUKADA, T., and Y. KAWADE: Chromatography of ribonucleic acid of high molecular weight isolated from FL cells infected with ECHO 7 virus. Virology 19, 409 (1963).

GAILBRAITH, N. S.: A survey of enteroviruses and adenoviruses in the feces of normal children aged 0—4 years. J. Hyg. (Lond.) 63, 441 (1965).

GALPINE, J. F., T. M. CLAYTON, J. ARDLEY, and N. BASTER: Outbreak of aseptic meningitis with exanthem. Brit. med. J. 1, 319 (1958).

GAUDIN, G., A. M. BARRAL et R. SOHIER: Hémagglutination par certains types de virus ECHO 1. Etude de quelques caractères des hémagglutinines. Ann. Inst. Pasteur 104, 313 (1963).

GEAR, J. H. S.: Personal communication cited by EGGERS and SABIN (1959).

GELFAND, H. M.: The occurrence in nature of the Coxsackie and ECHO viruses. Progr. med. Virol. 3, 193 (1961).

GELFAND, H. M., J. P. FOX, and D. R. LEBLANC: The enteric viral flora of a population of normal children in southern Louisiana. Amer. J. trop. Med. Hyg. 6, 521 (1957).

GELFAND, H. M., A. H. HOLGUIN, G. E. MARCHETTI, and P. M. FEORINO: A continuing surveillance of enterovirus infections in healthy children in six United States cities. 1. Viruses isolated during 1960 and 1961. Amer J. Hyg. 78, 358 (1963).

GNESH, M., H. PLAGER, and W. DECHER: Enterovirus typing by complement fixation. Proc. Soc. exp. Biol. (N.Y.) 115, 898 (1964).

GODMAN, G. C., R. A. RIFKIND, C. HOWE. and H. M. ROSE: A description of ECHO 9 virus infection in cultured cells. I. The cytopathic effect. Amer. J. Path. 44, 1 (1964a).

GODMAN, G. C., R. A. RIFKIND, R. B. PAGE, C. HOWE, and H. M. ROSE: A description of ECHO-9 virus infection in cultured cells. II. Cytochemical observations. Amer. J. Path. 44, 215 (1964b).

GODTFREDSEN, A.: Typing of freshly isolated strains of polio, ECHO and Coxsackie viruses by complement fixation. Acta path. microbiol. scand. 49, 189 (1960).

GODTFREDSEN, A., and H. VON MAGNUS: Isolation of ECHO virus type 9 from cerebrospinal fluids. Dan. med. Bull. 4, 233 (1957).

GOLDFIELD, M., S. SRIHONGSE, and J. P. FOX: Hemagglutinins associated with certain human enteric viruses. Proc. Soc. exp. Biol. (N.Y.) 96, 788 (1957).

GOULET, N. R., K. W. COCHRAN, and G. C. BROWN: Differential and specific inhibition of ECHO viruses by plant extracts. Proc. Soc. exp. Biol. (N.Y.) 103, 96 (1960).

GREEN, M.: Chemistry and structure of animal viruses. Amer. J. Med. 38, 651 (1965).

GRIST, N. R., and E. J. BELL: ECHO 7 virus infections in Scotland. Letter to the editor. Brit. med. J. 2, 504 (1963).

GUERIN, L. F., and M. M. GUERIN: Susceptibility of pig kidney tissue cultures to certain viruses. Proc. Soc. exp. Biol. (N.Y.) 96, 322 (1957).

HABEL, K., J. W. HORNIBROOK, N. C. GREGG, R. J. SILVERBERG, and K. K. TAKEMOTO: The effect of anticellular sera on virus multiplication in tissue culture. Virology 5, 7 (1958).

HALONEN, P., and R. J. HUEBNER: ECHO and poliomyelitis virus antisera prepared in guinea pigs with fluorocarbon treated cell culture antigens. Proc. Soc. exp. Biol. (N.Y.) 105, 46 (1960).

HALONEN, P., R. J. HUEBNER, and C. TURNER: Preparation of ECHO complement-fixing antigens in monkey kidney tissue culture and their purification by fluorocarbon. Proc. Soc. exp. Biol. (N.Y.) 97, 530 (1958).

HALONEN, P., L. ROSEN, and R. J. HUEBNER: Typing of ECHO viruses by a complement fixation technic. Proc. Soc. exp. Biol. (N.Y.) 98, 105 (1958).

HALONEN, P., L. ROSEN, and R. J. HUEBNER: Homologous and heterologous complement fixing antibody in persons infected with ECHO, Coxsackie and polioviruses. Proc. Soc. exp. Biol. (N.Y.) 101, 236 (1959).

HALPEREN, S., H. J. EGGERS, and I. TAMM: Evidence for uncoupled synthesis of viral RNA and viral capsids. Virology 24, 36 (1964a).

HALPEREN, S., H. J. EGGERS, and I. TAMM: Complete and coreless hemagglutinating particles produced in ECHO 12 virus-infected cells. Virology 23, 81 (1964b).

HAMBLING, M. H., and P. M. DAVIS: Susceptibility of the LLC-MK₂ line of monkey kidney cells to human enteroviruses. J. Hyg. (Lond.) 63, 169 (1965).

HAMMON, W. McD., E. H. LUDWIG, G. E. SATHER, and W. D. SCHRACK, Jr.: A longitudinal study of infection with poliomyelitis viruses in American families on a Philippine military base, during an interepidemic period. Ann. N.Y. Acad. Sci. 61, 979 (1955).

HAMMON, W. McD., E. H. LUDWIG, G. SATHER, and D. S. YOHN: Comparative studies on patterns of family infections with polioviruses and ECHO virus type 1 on an American military base in the Philippines. Amer. J. publ. Hlth 47, 802 (1957).

HAMMON, W. McD., D. S. YOHN, E. H. LUDWIG, R. A. PAVIA, G. E. SATHER, and L. W. MCCLOSKEY: A study of certain nonpoliomyelitis and poliomyelitis enterovirus infections. J. Amer. med. Ass. 167, 727 (1958).

HAMMON, W. McD., D. S. YOHN, and R. A. PAVIA: ECHO virus type 12, isolation and characteristics. Proc. Soc. exp. Biol. (N.Y.) **100,** 743 (1959).

HAMMON, W. McD., D. S. YOHN, R. A. PAVIA, and G. SATHER: ECHO virus type 13. I. Isolation and characteristics. Proc. Soc. exp. Biol. (N.Y.) **100.** 425 (1959).

HAMMON, W. McD., D. S. YOHN, R. A. PAVIA, and G. E. SATHER: ECHO virus type 13. II. Epidemiologic aspects and clinical associations. Amer. J. trop. Med. Hvg. **10,** 62 (1961).

HAMPIL, B., J. L. MELNICK, C. WALLIS, R. W. BROWN, E. T. BRAYE, and R. R. ADAMS, Jr.: Preparation of antiserum to enteroviruses in large animals. J. Immunol. **95,** 895 (1965).

HANZON, V., and L. PHILIPSON: Ultrastructure and spatial arrangement of ECHO virus particles in purified preparations. J. Ultrastruct. Res. **3,** 420 (1960).

HAYFLICK, L., and P. S. MOORHEAD: The serial cultivation of human diploid cell strains. Exp. Cell Res. **25,** 585 (1961).

HENIGST, W. W., H. M. GELFAND, D. R. LEBLANC, and J. P. FOX: ECHO virus type 7 infections in continuously observed population group in Southern Louisiana. Amer. J. trop. Med. Hyg. **10,** 759 (1961).

HIATT, C. W., E. KAUFMAN, J. J. HELPRIN, and S. BARON: Inactivation of viruses by the photodynamic action of toluidine blue. J. Immunol. **84,** 480 (1960).

HINUMA, Y., K. URUNO, M. MORITA, N. ISHIDA, and T. NAKAO: Virological and epidemiological studies of an outbreak of aseptic meningitis caused by ECHO virus 4 in northern Japan in 1964. J. Hyg. (Lond.) **64,** 53 (1966).

HOLLAND, J. J.: Irreversible eclipse of poliovirus by HeLa cells. Virology **16,** 163 (1962).

HOLLAND, J. J., and B. H. HOYER: Early stages of enterovirus infection. Cold Spr. Harb. Symp. quant. Biol. **27,** 101 (1962).

HOLLAND, J. J., L. C. McLAREN, and J. G. SYVERTON: The mammalian cell virus relationship. IV. Infection of naturally insusceptible cells with enterovirus ribonucleic acid. J. exp. Med. **110,** 65 (1959).

HORSTMANN, D. M.: The new ECHO viruses and their role in human disease. Arch. intern. Med. **102,** 155 (1958).

HOYER, B. H., E. T. BOLTON, R. A. ORMSBEE, G. LEBOUVIER, D. B. RITTER, and C. LARSON: Mammalian viruses and rickettsiae. Their purification and recovery by cellulose anion exchange columns has significant implications. Science **127,** 859 (1958).

HSIUNG, G. D.: Further studies on characterization and grouping of ECHO viruses. Ann. N.Y. Acad. Sci. **101,** 413 (1962).

HSIUNG, G. D., and J. L. MELNICK: Morphologic characteristics of plaques produced on monkey kidney monolayer cultures by enteric viruses (poliomyelitis, Coxsackie and ECHO groups). J. Immunol. **78,** 128 (1957a).

HSIUNG, G. D., and J. L. MELNICK: Comparative susceptibility of kidney cells from different monkey species to enteric viruses (poliomyelitis, Coxsackie, and ECHO groups). J. Immunol. **78,** 137 (1957b).

HULL, R. N., W. R. CHERRY, and O. J. TRITCH: Growth characteristics of monkey kidney cell strains LLC-MK$_1$, and LLC-MK$_2$ (NCTC-3196) and their utility in virus research. J. exp. Med. **115,** 903 (1962).

ITOH, H., and J. L. MELNICK: The infection of chimpanzees with ECHO viruses. J. exp. Med. **106,** 677 (1957).

JAMISON, R. M., and H. D. MAYOR: Comparative study of seven picornaviruses of man. J. Bact. **91,** 1971 (1966).

JAMISON, R. M., H. D. MAYOR, and J. L. MELNICK: Studies on ECHO 4 virus (picornavirus group) and its intracellular development. Exp. molec. Path. **2,** 188 (1963).

JOHNSON, R. T., B. PORTNOY, N. G. ROGERS, and E. L. BUESCHER: Acute benign pericarditis. Virologic study of 34 patients. Arch. intern. Med. **108,** 823 (1961).

JOHNSON, T.: A new clinical entity? Lancet **272,** 590 (1957).

JOHNSSON, T., M. BÖTTIGER, and A. LÖFDAHL: An outbreak of aseptic meningitis with a rubella-like rash probably caused by ECHO virus type 4. Arch. ges. Virusforsch. 8, 306 (1958).

JOHNSSON, T., B. JÖNSSON, E. LYCKE, and B. WICTORIN: Studies on an epidemic of aseptic meningitis associated with Coxsackie and ECHO viruses. Arch. ges. Virusforsch. 7, 384 (1957).

JOHNSSON, T., B. LYCKE, B. WICTORIN, and B. JÖNSSON: Studies of an epidemic of aseptic meningitis in association with Coxsackie and ECHO viruses. II. Serological and clinical observations. Arch. ges. Virusforsch. 8, 285 (1958).

JOKLIK, W. K., and J. E. DARNEL, Jr.: The adsorption and early fate of purified poliovirus in HeLa cells. Virology 13, 439 (1961).

JORDAN, W. S.: Newer viruses. DM (Disease-a-Month) page 1 (1959).

KABLER, P. W., N. A. CLARKE, G. BERG, and L. CHANG: Viricidal efficiency of disinfectants in water. Publ. Hlth Rep. (Wash.) 76, 565 (1961).

KALTER, S. S.: A serological survey of antibodies to selected enteroviruses. Bull. Wld Hlth Org. 26, 759 (1962).

KALTER, S. S., R. FUENTES-MARINS, A. R. RODRIGUEZ, A. HELLMAN, R. A. CRANDELL, and N. T. WERTHESSEN: Susceptibility of baboon (Papio doguera) kidney cells to human enteroviruses. Proc. Soc. exp. Biol. (N.Y.) 111, 337 (1962).

KAMITSUKA, P. S., M. E. SOERGEL, and H. A. WENNER: Production and standardization of ECHO reference antisera. I. For 25 prototypic ECHO viruses. Amer. J. Hyg. 74, 7 (1961).

KANTOR, F. S., and G. D. HSIUNG: Pleurodynia associated with ECHO virus type 8. New Engl. J. Med. 266, 661 (1962).

KARZON, D. T., A. L. BARRON, W. WINKELSTEIN, Jr., and S. COHEN: Isolation of ECHO virus type 6 during outbreak of seasonal aseptic meningitis. J. Amer. med. Ass. 162, 1298 (1956).

KARZON, D. T., G. L. ECKERT, A. L. BARRON, N. S. HAYNER, and W. WINKELSTEIN: Aseptic meningitis epidemic due to ECHO 4 virus. Amer. J. Dis. Child. 101, 610 (1961).

KARZON, D. T., N. S. HAYNER, W. WINKELSTEIN, Jr., and A. L. BARRON: An epidemic of aseptic meningitis syndrome due to ECHO virus type 6. II. A clinical study of ECHO 6 infection. Pediatrics 29, 418 (1962).

KARZON, D. T., B. F. POLLOCK, and A. L. BARRON: Phase variation in ECHO virus type 6. Virology 9, 564 (1959).

KASEL. J. A., L. ROSEN, F. LODA, and W. FLEET: ECHO virus type 25, infection in adult volunteers. Proc. Soc. exp. Biol. (N.Y.) 118, 381 (1965).

KAVELMAN. D. A., I. B. R. DUNCAN, and J. A. LEWIS: Acute benign pericarditis. Canad. med. Ass. J. 85, 1287 (1961).

KAWANA*, R.: An epidemic of aseptic meningitis due to ECHO virus 6. Med. Biol. (Tokyo) 71, 356 (1965).

KAWANA*, R., et al.: Epidemic of aseptic meningitis due to ECHO virus 4. Epidemic breakout in the town of Karumai-Cho, Iwati Prefecture in 1964. Med. Biol. (Tokyo) 71, 296 (1965).

KELLY, S.: Enteric virus isolation from sewage. Acta med. scand. 159, 63 (1957).

KELLY, S., and W. W. SANDERSON: Enteric viruses in wading pools. Publ. Hlth Rep. (Wash.) 76, 199 (1961).

KERN, J., and L. ROSEN: Factors affecting hemagglutination by enteroviruses. Proc. Soc. exp. Biol. (N. Y.) 115, 536 (1964).

KIBRICK, S.: Current status of Coxsackie and ECHO viruses in human disease. Progr. med. Virol. 6, 27 (1964).

KIBRICK, S., and J. F. ENDERS: (cited by T. H. WELLER) The application of tissue culture methods to the studies of polyomyelitis. New Engl. J. Med. 249, 186 (1953).

KIBRICK, S., L. MELENDEZ, and J. F. ENDERS: Clinical associations of enteric viruses with particular reference to agents exhibiting properties of the ECHO group. Ann. N.Y. Acad. Sci. 67, 311 (1957).

KING, D. L., and D. T. KARZON: An epidemic of aseptic meningitis syndrome due to ECHO virus type 6. III. Sequelae three years after infection. Pediatrics **29,** 432 (1962).

KITANO, T., I. HARUNA, and I. WATANABE: Purification and concentration of viruses by an organic solvent system. Virology **15,** 503 (1961).

KLEIN, J. O., A. M. LERNER, and M. FINLAND: Acute gastroenteritis associated with ECHO virus, type 11. Amer. J. med. Sci. **240,** 749 (1960).

KLEINMAN, H., M. K. COONEY, C. B. NELSON, R. R. OWEN, L. BOYD, and G. SWANDA: Aseptic meningitis and paralytic disease due to newly recognized enteroviruses. J. Amer. med. Ass. **187,** 90 (1964).

KLEINMAN, H., D. G. RAMRAS, M. K. COONEY, and L. BOYD: Aseptic meningitis due to ECHO virus type 7. New Engl. J. Med. **267,** 1116 (1962).

KLEINMAN, H., D. ROGERS, P. M. ELIWOOD, H. BRUHL, L. M. SCHUMAN, and H. BAUER: Epidemic of ECHO 9 aseptic meningitis in Minnesota, 1957. Univ. Minn. med. Bull. **29,** 306 (1958).

KON*, A., et al.: Aseptic meningitis caused by ECHO 4. Acta Paed. (Japan) **69,** 513 (1965).

KONO, R., C. HAMADA, M. HOSINO, T. FUKADA, Y. ASHIHARA, and H. YAOI, Jr.: Studies on mixed infection with poliovirus type 1 and ECHO virus type 7 in monkeys and cell cultures. Amer. J. Hyg. 78, 89 (1963).

KOPEL, F. B., B. SHORE, and H. L. HODES: Nonfatal bulbospinal paralysis due to ECHO 4 virus. J. Pediat. **67,** 588 (1965).

KRECH, U.: Über das Vorkommen von ECHO-Virus in der Schweiz. Schweiz. med. Wschr. **87,** 1 (1957).

KUNIN, C. M.: Virus-tissue union and the pathogenesis of enterovirus infections. J. Immunol. **88,** 556 (1962).

LAFOREST, R. A., G. A. McNAUGHTON, A. J. BEALE, M. CLARKE, M. DAVIS, L. SULTANIAN, and A. J. RHODES: Outbreak of aseptic meningitis (meningoencephalitis) with rubelliform rash. Toronto, 1956. Canad. med. Ass. J. **77,** 1 (1957).

LAHELLE, O.: Multiplication of poliomyelitis and ECHO viruses in tissue cultures prepared from human amniotic membranes. Acta path. microbiol. scand. **40,** 436 (1957).

LAHELLE, O.: Capacity of certain ECHO virus 6 strains to cause hemagglutination. Virology **5,** 110 (1958a).

LAHELLE, O.: Inhibition of ECHO virus hemagglutination by specific ECHO antisera. Acta path. microbiol. scand. **44,** 413 (1958b).

LAMB, G. A., T. D. Y. CHIN, and L. E. SCARCE: Isolations of enteric viruses from sewage and river water in a metropolitan area. Amer. J. Hyg. 80, 320 (1964).

LAMB, R. D., and G. R. DUBES: Chromatography of enteroviral ribonucleic acids on hydromagnesite. Analyt. Biochem. **7,** 152 (1964).

LANDSMAN, J. B., et al.: Poliomyelitis-like disease in 1959. A combined Scottish study. Brit. med. J. **2,** 597 (1961).

LAPINLEIMU, K., and K. PENTTINEN: Virus isolations from sewage in Finland in 1960—1961. Arch. ges. Virusforsch. **13,** 72 (1963).

LEE, L. H., C. A. PHILLIPS, M. A. SOUTH, J. L. MELNICK, and M. D. YOW: Enteric virus isolation in different cell cultures. Bull. Wld Hlth Org. **32,** 657 (1965).

LEHAN, P. H., E. W. CHICK, I. L. DOTO, T. D. Y. CHIN, R. H. HEEREN, and M. L. FURCOLOW: An epidemic illness associated with a recently recognized enteric virus (ECHO virus type 4). I. Epidemiologic and clinical features. Amer. J. Hyg. **66,** 63 (1957).

LEHMANN-GRUBE, F.: Cooperative susceptibility of mammalian cells in culture to prototype enteroviruses. Arch. ges. Virusforsch. **11,** 276 (1961).

LEHMANN-GRUBE, F., and J. T. SYVERTON: Thermal inactivation of ECHO viruses in cell culture medium. Amer. J. Hyg. **69,** 161 (1959).

LENAHAN, M. F., and H. A. WENNER: Propagation of entero- and other viruses in renal cells obtained from non-primate hosts. J. infect. Dis. **107,** 203 (1960).

LENNETTE, E. H., N. J. SCHMIDT, and R. L. MAGOFFIN: Observations on the complement-fixing antibody response to poliovirus in patients with certain Coxsackie and ECHO virus infections. J. Immunol. **86**, 552 (1961).

LENNETTE, E. H., N. J. SCHMIDT, R. L. MAGOFFIN, J. DENNIS, and A. WIENER: The Price virus. An unclassified enterovirus isolated from patients with central nervous system disease. Proc. Soc. exp. Biol. (N.Y.) **110**, 769 (1962).

LENNETTE, E. H., N. J. SCHMIDT, R. L. MAGOFFIN, S. J. HAGENS, and E. J. DUKELLIS: A comparison of the reactivity of poliovirus complement-fixing antigens (native, heated and sucrose density gradient C and D) with human sera. J. Immunol. **92**, 261 (1964).

LÉPINE, P., J. SAMAILLE, J. MAURIN, O. DUBOIS et M. C. CARRÉ: Isolement du virus ECHO 14 au cours d'une épidémie de créche de gastro-entéritis. Ann. Inst. Pasteur **99**, 161 (1960).

LEPOW, M. L., N. COYNE, L. B. THOMPSON, D. H. CARVER, and F. C. ROBBINS: A clinical epidemiologic and laboratory investigation of aseptic meningitis during the four-year period, 1955—1958. II. The clinical disease and its sequelae. New Engl. J. Med. **266**, 1188 (1962).

LERNER, A. M., E. J. BAILEY, and J. R. TILLOTSON: Enterovirus hemagglutination: Inhibition by several enzymes and sugars. J. Immunol. **95**, 1111 (1966a).

LERNER, A. M., L. D. GELB, J. R. TILLOTSON, M. M. CARRUTHERS, and E. J. BAILEY: Enterovirus hemagglutination: Inhibition by aldoses and a possible mechanism. J. Immunol. **96**, 629 (1966b).

LI, C. P.: Experimental variation in mouse virulence of ECHO 9 virus. Proc. Soc. exp. Biol. (N.Y.) **102**, 233 (1959).

LIEBHABER, H., and K. K. TAKEMOTO: The basis for the size differences on plaques produced by variants of encephalomyocarditis (EMC) virus. Virology **20**, 559 (1963).

LIM, K. A., and M. BENYESH-MELNICK: Typing of viruses by combinations of antiserum pools. Application to typing of enteroviruses (Coxsackie and ECHO). J. Immunol. **84**, 309 (1960).

LOU, T. Y., and H. A. WENNER: Experimental infection with enteroviruses. V. Studies on virulence and pathogenesis in cynomolgus monkeys. Arch. ges. Virusforsch. **12**, 303 (1962).

LUND, E.: Oxidative inactivation of different types of enteroviruses. Amer. J. Hyg. **80**, 1 (1964).

LUND, E., and C.-E. HEDSTRÖM: The use of an aqueous polymer phase system for enterovirus isolations from sewage. Amer. J. Epidem. **84**, 287 (1966).

LUND, E., C.-E. HEDSTRÖM, and O. STRANNEGÅRD: A comparison between virus isolations from sewage and from fecal specimens from patients. Amer. J. Epidem. **84**, 282 (1966).

LWOFF, A.: The concept of virus. J. gen. Microbiol. **17**, 239 (1957).

LWOFF, A., and P. TOURNIER: The classification of viruses. Ann. Rev. Microbiol. **20**, 45 (1966).

McALLISTER, R. M., K. HUMMELER, and L. L. CORIELL: Acute cerebellar ataxia. Report of a case with isolation of type 9 ECHO virus from the cerebrospinal fluid. New Engl. J. Med. **261**, 1159 (1959).

McINTOSH, E. G. S., and R. G. SOMMERVILLE: An analysis of 24 strains of ECHO virus type 7. Arch. ges. Virusforsch. **9**, 261 (1959).

McLAREN, L. C., J. J. HOLLAND, and J. T. SYVERTON: The mammalian cell-virus relationship. I. Attachment of poliovirus to cultivated cells of primate and nonprimate origin. J. exp. Med. **109**, 475 (1959).

McLEAN, D. M.: Infection hazards in swimming pools. Pediatrics **31**, 811 (1963).

McLEAN, D. M., and J. L. MELNICK: Association of mouse pathogenic strain of ECHO virus type 9 with aseptic meningitis. Proc. Soc. exp. Biol. (N.Y.) **94**, 656 (1957).

MAISEL, J., and C. MOSCOVICI: Plaque formation with ECHO virus types 15 to 24. J. Immunol. **86**, 635 (1961).

MAISEL, J., C. MOSCOVICI, and M. LAPLACA: Susceptibility of human tumor cells to ECHO viruses and loss of hemagglutinating capacity of some of the adapted viruses. Arch. ges. Virusforsch. **11**, 209 (1961).

MAJIMA*, E., et al.: A paralytic patient with a condition similar to the spinal form of poliomyelitis and with ECHO 4 type virus in the spinal fluid. Acta Pediat. (Japan) **69**, 295 (1965).

MALHERBE, H., R. HARWIN, and A. H. SMITH: An outbreak of aseptic meningitis associated with ECHO virus type 4. S. Afr. med. J. **31**, 1261 (1957).

MATUMOTO, M.: Newer respiratory disease viruses in Japan and some for Eastern countries. Conference on Newer Respiratory Disease Viruses, Bethesda, 1962. Amer. Rev. resp. Dis., pp. 46 (1962).

MAYER, M. M., H. J. RAPP, B. ROIZMAN, S. W. KLEIN, K. M. COWAN, D. LUKENS, C. E. SCHWERDT, F. L. SCHAFFER, and J. CHARNEY: The purification of poliomyelitis virus as studied by complement fixation. J. Immunol. **78**, 435 (1957).

MAYOR, H. D.: Picornavirus symmetry. Discussion and preliminary reports. Virology **22**, 156 (1964).

MEDEARIS, D. N., Jr., and R. A. KRAMER: Exanthem associated with ECHO virus type 18 viremia. J. Pediat. **55**, 367 (1959).

MELNICK, J. L.: Application of tissue culture methods to epidemiological studies of poliomyelitis. Amer. J. publ. Hlth **44**, 571 (1954).

MELNICK, J. L.: ECHO viruses. Special publication. N.Y. Acad. Sci. **5**, 365 (1957).

MELNICK, J. L.: Advances in the study of enteroviruses. Progr. med. Virol. **1**, 59 (1958).

MELNICK, J. L.: Enteroviruses. Ann. N.Y. Acad. Sci. **101**, 331 (1962).

MELNICK, J. L.: Chairman, International Enterovirus Study Group: Picornavirus group. Virology **19**, 114 (1963).

MELNICK, J. L., G. DALLDORF, J. F. ENDERS, H. M. GELFAND, W. McD. HAMMON, R. J. HUEBNER, L. ROSEN, A. B. SABIN, J. T. SYVERTON, and H. A. WENNER: Classification of human enteroviruses. Virology **16**, 501 (1962).

MELNICK, J. L., J. EMMONS, J. H. COFFEY, and H. SCHOOF: Seasonal distribution of Coxsackie viruses in urban sewage and flies. Amer. J. Hyg. **59**, 164 (1954).

MELNICK, J. L., and B. HAMPIL: WHO collaborative studies on enterovirus reference antisera. Bull. Wld Hlth Org. **33**, 761 (1965).

MELNICK, J. L., and R. M. McCOMBS: Classification and nomenclature of animal viruses. Progr. med. Virol. **8**, 400 (1966).

MELNICK, J. L., H. A. WENNER, and L. ROSEN: Enteroviruses. Diagnostic Procedures for Viral and Rickettsial Diseases, 3rd ed. Amer. publ. Hlth Ass., p. 194 (1964).

Microbiological Associates, Inc.: Statement concerning the preparation and use of ECHO virus antisera for types 1 to 14 and Coxsackie virus antisera for types B1 to B5 and A9 (1957).

MIDDLETON, G. K., Jr., H. G. CRAMBLETT, H. L. MOFFET, J. P. BLACK, and H. SHULENBERGER: Micro diffusion precipitin tests for enteroviruses and influenza B virus. J. Bact. **87**, 1171 (1964).

MIDULLA, M., C. WALLIS, and J. L. MELNICK: Enterovirus immunizing antigens in the form of cation-stabilized and concentrated virus preparations. J. Immunol. **95**, 9 (1965).

MONTAGNIER, L., and F. K. SANDERS: Replicative form of encephalomyocarditis virus ribonucleic acid. Nature (Lond.) **199**, 664 (1963).

MOORE, M. L., L. E. HOOSER, E. V. DAVIS, and R. A. SIEM: Sudden unexpected death in infancy. Isolations of ECHO type 7 virus. Proc. Soc. exp. Biol. (N.Y.) **116**, 231 (1964).

MOSCOVICI, C., A. GINEVRI, and C. H. KEMPE: The distribution of poliomyelitis and ECHO viruses in a children's institution. Amer. J. Dis. Child. **98**, 139 (1959).

NEVA, F. A.: A second outbreak of Boston exanthem disease in Pittsburgh during 1954. New Engl. J. Med. **254**, 838 (1956).

NEVA, F. A., and J. F. ENDERS: Cytopathic agents isolated from patients during an unusual epidemic exanthem. J. Immunol. **72**, 307 (1954).

NEVA, F. A., R. F. FEEMSTER, and I. J. GORBACH: Clinical and epidemiological features of an unusual epidemic exanthem. J. Amer. med. Ass. **155**, 544 (1954).

NEVA, F. A., and M. F. MALONE: Specific and cross reactions by complement fixation with Boston exanthem disease virus (ECHO-16). J. Immunol. **83**, 645 (1959a).

NEVA, F. A., and M. F. MALONE: Persistence of antibodies to ECHO-16 viruses following Boston exanthem disease. Proc. Soc. exp. Biol. (N.Y.) **102**, 233 (1959b).

NEVA, F. A., M. F. MALONE, and L. J. LEWIS: Antigenic comparison of Boston exanthem virus strains and their relationship to ECHO-16 virus as studied by neutralization and complement fixation procedure. J. Immunol. **83**, 653 (1959).

NIHOUL, E., L. QUERSIN-THIRY, and A. WEYNANTS: ECHO virus type 9 as the agent responsible for an important outbreak of aseptic meningitis in Belgium. Amer. J. Hyg. **66**, 102 (1957).

NÚÑEZ-MONTIEL, O., J. WEIBEL, and J. VITELLI-FLORES: Electron microscopic study of the cytopathology of ECHO virus infection in cultivated cells. J. biophys. biochem. Cytol. **11**, 457 (1961).

OCAMPO, A. R., and J. L. MELNICK: Production of high-titer enterovirus antisera in baboons. Amer. J. Hyg. **79**, 349 (1964).

OZERES, R. L., R. FAULKNER, and C. E. VAN ROOYEN: Enteroviruses in sewage and epidemic poliomyelitis in Eastern Canada. Canad. med. Ass. J. **85**, 1419 (1961).

PAFFENBARGER, R. S., Jr., G. BERG, N. A. CLARKE, R. E. STEVENSON, B. G. POOLER, and R. T. HYDE: Viruses and illnesses in a boy's summer camp. Amer. J. Hyg. **70**, 254 (1959).

PAL, S. R., J. McQUILLEN, and P. S. GARDNER: A comparative study of susceptibility of primary monkey kidney cells, HEp-2 cells and HeLa cells to a variety of faecal viruses. J. Hyg. (Lond.) **61**, 493 (1963).

PARKS, W. P., J. L. MELNICK, L. T. QUEIROGA, and H. ALI KHAN: Studies of infantile diarrhea in Karachi, Pakistan. I. Collection, virus isolation and typing of viruses. Amer. J. Epidem. **84**, 382 (1966).

PETTE, H., G. MAASS, L. VALENCIANO und K. MANNWEILER: Zur Frage der Neuropathogenität von Enteroviren. Experimentelle Untersuchungen zur Neuropathogenität verschiedener Stämme von ECHO-9 Virus. Arch. ges. Virusforsch. **10**, 408 (1961).

PHILIPSON, L.: Recovery of a cytopathogenic agent from patients with non-diphtheritic croup and from day-nursery children. III. Studies on the hemagglutination and hemagglutination-inhibition of the agent. Arch. ges. Virusforsch. **8**, 332 (1958).

PHILIPSON, L., P. Å. ALBERTSSON, and G. FRICK: The purification and concentration of viruses by aqueous polymer phase systems. Virology **11**, 553 (1960).

PHILIPSON, L., and S. BENGTSSON: Interaction of enteroviruses with receptors from erythrocytes and host cells. Virology **18**, 457 (1962).

PHILIPSON, L., S. BENGTSSON, S. BRISHAMMAR, L. SVENNERHOLM, and Ö. ZETTERQVIST: Purification and chemical analysis of the erythrocytic receptor for hemagglutinating enteroviruses. Virology **22**, 580 (1964).

PHILIPSON, L., and P. W. CHOPPIN: On the role of virus sulfhydryl groups in the attachment of enteroviruses to erythrocytes. J. exp. Med. **112**, 445 (1960).

PHILIPSON, L., and P. W. CHOPPIN: Inactivation of enteroviruses by 2,3-Dimercaptopropanol (BAL). Virology **16**, 405 (1962).

PHILIPSON, L., and M. LIND: Enterovirus eclipse in a cell-free system. Virology **23**, 322 (1964).

PHILIPSON, L., and L. ROSEN: Identification of a cytopathogenic agent called U-virus recovered from patients with non-diphtheritic croup and from day nursery children. Arch. ges. Virusforsch. **9**, 25 (1959).

PINDAK, F. F., and W. E. CLAPPER: Isolation of enteric cytopathogenic human orphan virus type 6 from dogs. Amer. J. vet. Res. **25**, 52 (1964).

PINDAK, F. F., and W. E. CLAPPER: Experimental infection of beagles with ECHO virus type 6. AEC Research and Development Report, Lovelace Foundation, Albuquerque, New Mexico (1965).

PINDAK, F. F., and W. E. CLAPPER: Experimental infection of beagles with ECHO virus type 6. Tex. Rep. Biol. Med. 24, 468 (1966).

PLAGER, H., and F. F. HARRISON: Paralysis associated with ECHO virus type 9. N.Y. St. J. Med. 61, 798 (1961).

PLUMMER, G.: The picornaviruses of man and animals. A comparative review. Progr. med. Virol. 7, 326 (1965).

PODOPLEKIN, V. D.: Studies on the hemagglutinating properties of ECHO viruses. Acta virol. 7, 131 (1963).

PODOPLEKIN, V. D.: Effect of tissue cultures on the hemagglutinating properties of ECHO viruses and mechanism of the interaction of these viruses with erythrocytes. Acta virol. 8, 254 (1964).

PODOPLEKIN, V. D., and T. I. IVANOVA: Some intratypic differences between hemagglutinating ECHO viruses. Acta virol. 9, 397 (1965).

PODOPLEKIN, V. D., and T. I. IVANOVA: Stabilization of ECHO virus haemagglutinins. I. Thermal inactivation of haemagglutinins and their cationic stabilization. Acta virol. 10, 89 (1966).

PODOPLEKIN, V. D., and E. M. NOVYSH: Stabilization of ECHO virus haemagglutinins. II. Stabilization with organic compounds. Acta virol. 10, 97 (1966).

PODOPLEKIN, V. D., E. M. NOVYSH, and L. E. PODOPLEKINA: Stabilization of ECHO virus haemagglutinins. III. Some peculiarities of the stabilization with organic compounds. Acta virol. 10, 248 (1966).

POHJANPELTO, P.: Response of enteroviruses to cystine. Virology 15, 225 (1961).

POLSON, A., and D. DEEKS: Zone electrophoresis of enteroviruses. J. Hyg. (Lond.) 60, 217 (1962).

PONS, M.: Infectious double-stranded poliovirus RNA. Virology 24, 467 (1964).

QUERSIN-THIRY, L.: Action of anticellular sera on virus infections. I. Influence on homologous tissue cultures infected with various viruses. J. Immunol. 81, 253 (1958).

RAMOS-ALVAREZ, M., F. GOMEZ-SANTOS, L. RONGEL-RIVERA, and O. MAYES: Viral and serological studies of children immunized with oral poliovirus vaccine — preliminary report of a large trial conducted in Mexico. International Conference on Live Poliovirus Vaccines. 1st. (Scientific Publication No. 44, Pan American Sanitary Bureau.) Washington, D. C., pp. 483 (1959).

RAMOS-ALVAREZ, M., and J. OLARTE: Diarrheal diseases of children. The occurrence of enteropathogenic viruses and bacteria. Amer. J. Dis. Child. 107, 218 (1964).

RAMOS-ALVAREZ, M., and A. B. SABIN: Characteristics of poliovirus and other enteric viruses recovered in tissue culture from healthy American children. Proc. Soc. exp. Biol. (N.Y.) 87, 655 (1954).

RAMOS-ALVAREZ, M., and A. B. SABIN: Enteropathogenic viruses and bacteria: Role in summer diarrheal diseases of infancy and early childhood. J. Amer. med. Ass. 167, 147 (1958).

RAWLS, W. E., R. G. SHORTER, and E. C. HERRMANN, Jr.: Fatal neonatal illness associated with ECHO 9 (Coxsackie A 23) virus. Pediatrics 33, 278 (1964).

RAY, C. G., R. H. McCOLLOUGH, I. L. DOTO, J. C. TODD, W. P. GLEZEN, and T. D. Y. CHIN: ECHO 4 illness. Epidemiological, clinical and laboratory studies of an outbreak in a rural community. Amer. J. Epidem. 84, 253 (1966).

REILLY, C. M., J. STOKES, Jr., V. V. HAMPARIAN, and M. R. HILLEMAN: ECHO virus, type 25, in respiratory illness. J. Pediat. 62, 538 (1963).

REINHARD, K. R.: Ecology of enteroviruses in the Western Arctic. J. Amer. med. Ass. 183, 510 (1963).

RENDTORFF, R. C., L. C. WALKER, B. D. HALE, G. J. BILLMEIER, Jr., and A. N. ROBERTS: An epidemic of ECHO virus 2 infection in an orphanage nursery. Amer. J. Hyg. 79, 64 (1964).

RIFKIND, R. A., G. C. GODMAN, C. HOWE, C. MORGAN, and H. M. ROSE: Structure and development of viruses as observed in the electron microscope. VI. ECHO virus, type 9. J. exp. Med. 114, 1 (1961).

RIGGS, J. L., and G. C. BROWN: Application of direct and indirect immunofluorescence for identification of enteroviruses and titrating their antibodies. Proc. Soc. exp. Biol. (N.Y.) **110**, 833 (1962).

RIGHTSEL, W. A., J. R. DICE, R. J. MCALPINE, E. A. TIMM, I. W. MCLEAN, G. J. DIXON, and F. M. SCHABEL: Antiviral effect of guanidine. Science **134**, 558 (1961).

RIORDAN, J. T., R. J. PAUL, I. YOSHIOKA, and D. M. HORSTMANN: The detection of poliovirus and other enteric viruses in flies. Results of tests carried out during an oral poliovirus vaccine trial. Amer. J. Hyg. **74**, 123 (1961).

ROBBINS, F. C., J. F. ENDERS, T. H. WELLER, and G. L. FLORENTINO: Studies on the cultivation of poliomyelitis virus in tissue culture. V. The direct isolation and serologic identification of virus strains in tissue culture from patients with paralytic and nonparalytic poliomyelitis. Amer. J. Hyg. **54**, 286 (1951).

ROSEN, L.: Subclassification of picornaviruses. Bact. Rev. **29**, 173 (1965).

ROSEN, L., A. M. BEHBEHANI, P. S. KAMITSUKA, J. KERN, E. H. LENNETTE, J. L. MELNICK, N. J. SCHMIDT, and H. A. WENNER: On the alleged antigenic relationship between ECHO virus types 29 and 32. Proc. Soc. exp. Biol. (N.Y.) **119**, 908 (1965).

ROSEN, L., J. H. JOHNSON, R. J. HUEBNER, and J. A. BELL: Observations on a newly recognized ECHO virus and a description of an outbreak in a nursery. Amer. J. Hyg. **67**, 300 (1958).

ROSEN, L., J. KERN, and J. A. BELL: An outbreak of infection with ECHO virus type 3 associated with mild febrile illness. Amer. J. Hyg. **79**, 163 (1964).

ROTEM, C. E., and M. D. LAUSANNE: Meningitis of virus origin. Lancet **1**, 502 (1957).

ROUHANDEH, H.: Facilitation of infection of monkey kidney cells with certain picornavirus ribonucleic acids. Arch. ges. Virusforsch. **15**, 7 (1964).

ROUHANDEH, H., R. R. CHRONISTER, and M. L. BRINKMAN: Inhibition of poliovirus minute-plaque mutants and ECHO viruses by sulfated polysaccharides. Proc. Soc. exp. Biol. (N.Y.) **118**, 1118 (1965).

ROUHANDEH, H., and G. R. DUBES: Distinction of enteroviral ribonucleic acid infectivity by phosphodiesterase. Proc. Soc. exp. Biol. (N.Y.) **116**, 133 (1964).

ROUHANDEH, H., L. L. SELLS, and M. CHAPIN: Effect of L-cystine and sulfated polysaccharides on replication of ECHO virus type 32 in monkey kidney cells. Proc. Soc. exp. Biol. (N. Y.) **123**, 246 (1966).

SABIN, A. B.: Reoviruses. A new group of respiratory and enteric viruses formerly classified as ECHO type 10 is described. Science **130**, 1387 (1959).

SABIN, A. B., E. R. KRUMBIEGEL, and R. WIGAND: ECHO type 9 virus disease. Amer. J. Dis. Child. **96**, 197 (1958).

SABIN, A. B., M. RAMOS-ALVAREZ, W. ALVAREZ-AMÉZQUITA, R. H. PELON, et al.: Effects of rapid mass immunization of a population with live oral poliovirus vaccine under conditions of massive enteric infection with other viruses. In International Conference on Live Poliovirus Vaccines, 2nd. (Scientific Publication, No. 50, Pan American Health Organization.) Washington, D. C., pp. 377 (1960).

SACHTLEBEN, P., and K. MUNK: Some clinical findings in connection with ECHO type 6 virus infection. Mschr. Kinderheilk. **109**, 303 (1961).

SAKURADA, N., and A. M. PRINCE: Characteristics of disc assay for enterovirus antibody. Jap. J. exp. Med. **31**, 179 (1961).

SALZMAN, N. P., and E. D. SEBRING: The source of poliovirus ribonucleic acid. Virology **13**, 258 (1961).

SANFORD, J. P., and S. E. SULKIN: The clinical spectrum of ECHO-virus infection. New Engl. J. Med. **261**, 1113 (1959).

SCHAFFER, F. L., and L. H. FROMMHAGEN: Similarities of biophysical properties of several human enteroviruses as shown by density gradient ultracentrifugation of mixtures of the viruses. Virology **25**, 662 (1965).

SCHMIDT, N. J., J. DENNIS, S. J. HAGENS, and E. H. LENNETTE: Studies on hemagglutination and hemagglutination-inhibition tests for identification of ECHO viruses. Amer. J. Hyg. **75**, 74 (1962a).

SCHMIDT, N. J., J. DENNIS, S. J. HAGENS, and E. H. LENNETTE: Studies on the antibody responses of patients infected with ECHO viruses. Amer. J. Hyg. 75, 168 (1962b).

SCHMIDT, N. J., J. DENNIS, M. N. HOFFMAN, and E. H. LENNETTE: Inhibitors of ECHO virus and reovirus hemagglutination. I. Inhibitors in tissue culture fluids. J. Immunol. 93, 367 (1964a).

SCHMIDT, N. J., J. DENNIS, M. N. HOFFMAN, and E. H. LENNETTE: Inhibitors of ECHO virus and reovirus hemagglutination. II. Serum and phospholipid inhibitors. J. Immunol. 93, 377 (1964b).

SCHMIDT, N. J., J. DENNIS, and E. H. LENNETTE: Complement-fixing antibody responses to ECHO virus types 12 and 19 of patients with enterovirus infections. Proc. Soc. exp. Biol. (N.Y.) 109, 364 (1962).

SCHMIDT, N. J., J. DENNIS, and E. H. LENNETTE: Studies on filtrates from cultures of a psychrophilic *pseudomonas sp.* which inactivate nonspecific serum inhibitors for certain hemagglutinating viruses. J. Immunol. 93, 140 (1964).

SCHMIDT, N. J., R. W. GUENTHER, and E. H. LENNETTE: Typing of ECHO virus isolates by immune serum pools. The "intersecting serum scheme". J. Immunol. 87, 623 (1961).

SCHMIDT, N. J., H. H. HO, C. J. KING, J. DENNIS, and E. H. LENNETTE: Antigenic relationship between ECHO virus types 29 and 32. Proc. Soc. exp. Biol. (N.Y.) 116, 77 (1964d).

SCHMIDT, N. J., E. H. LENNETTE, J. H. DOLEMAN, and S. J. HAGENS: Factors influencing the potency of poliomyelitis complement-fixing antigens produced in tissue culture system. Amer. J. Hyg. 66, 1 (1957).

SCHMIDT, N. J., E. H. LENNETTE, and H. H. HO: Observations on antigenic variants of ECHO virus type 11. Proc. Soc. exp. Biol. (N. Y.) 123, 696 (1966).

SELWYN, S., and L. F. HOWITT: Mosaic of enteroviruses: poliovirus, Coxsackie and ECHO infections in group of families. Lancet 2, 548 (1962).

SELWYN, S., H. MONTGOMERY, and N. A. GRAY: Fatal illness associated with ECHO virus type 3 infection. Scot. med. J. 8, 162 (1963).

SHAVER, D. N., A. L. BARRON, and D. T. KARZON: Cytopathology of human enteric viruses in tissue culture. Amer. J. Path. 34, 943 (1958).

SHAVER, D. N., A. L. BARRON, and D. T. KARZON: Distinctive cytopathology of ECHO viruses types 22 and 23. Proc. Soc. exp. Biol. (N.Y.) 106, 648 (1961).

SHAW, E. D., A. NEWTON, A. W. POWELL, and C. J. FRIDAY: Fluorescent antigen-antibody reactions in Coxsackie and ECHO enteroviruses. Virology 15, 208 (1961).

SHINGU, M.: Studies on the complement fixation test with enteroviruses. Effects of heating antigens at various temperatures on their complement fixing ability. Kurume med. J. 8, 43 (1961).

SOLOMON, P., L. WEINSTEIN, TE-W. CHANG, M. S. ARTENSTEIN, and C. T. AMBROSE: Epidemiologic, clinical, and laboratory features of an epidemic of type 9 ECHO virus meningitis. J. Pediat. 55, 609 (1959).

SOMMERVILLE, R. G.: A microplaque method for counting enterovirus particles. Virology 9, 701 (1959).

SPIGLAND, I., J. P. FOX, L. R. ELVEBACK, F. E. WASSERMANN, A. KETLER, C. D. BRANDT, and A. KOGON: The virus watch program: A continuing surveillance of viral infections in metropolitan New York families. II. Laboratory methods and preliminary report on infections revealed by virus isolation. Amer. J. Epidem. 83, 413 (1966).

SPRUNT, K., W. M. REDMAN, and H. E. ALEXANDER: Infectious ribonucleic acid derived from enteroviruses. Proc. Soc. exp. Biol. (N.Y.) 101, 604 (1959).

STEIGMAN, A. J.: Poliomyelitic properties of certain nonpolioviruses: Enteroviruses and Heine-Medin disease. J. Mt Sinai Hosp. 25, 391 (1958).

STEIGMAN, A. J., and M. M. LIPTON: Fatal bulbospinal paralytic poliomyelitis due to ECHO 11 virus. J. Amer. med. Ass. 174, 178 (1960).

STUART, D. C., Jr., J. FOGH, and H. PLAGER: Cytoplasmic crystals in FL cells infected with an unclassified enteric virus (presumably a new type of ECHO virus). Virology 12, 321 (1960).

STULBERG, C. S., R. H. PAGE, and L. BERMAN: Comparative behavior of 16 ECHO virus types in fibroblast-like and epithelial-like human cell strains. Proc. Soc. exp. Biol. (N.Y.) 97, 355 (1958).

SUTO, T., D. T. KARZON, and R. H. BUSSELL: Studies of mutants of ECHO virus 6. III. Behavior in monkey and human cell culture. Amer. J. Epidem. 81, 341 (1965).

SUTO, T., D. T. KARZON, R. H. BUSSELL, and A. L. BARRON: Studies of mutants of ECHO virus 6. II. Isolation from human alimentary tract. Amer. J. Epidem. 81, 333 (1965).

TAKEMOTO, K. K., and H. LIEBHABER: Virus-polysaccharide interactions. I. An agar polysaccharide determining plaque morphology of EMC virus. Virology 14, 456 (1961).

TAMM, I., and H. J. EGGERS: Differences in the selective virus-inhibitory action of 2-(α-hydroxybenzyl)-benzimidazole and guanidine-HCl. Virology 18, 439 (1962).

TAMM, I., and H. J. EGGERS: Specific inhibition of replication of animal viruses. Science 142, 24 (1963).

TAMM, I., and H. J. EGGERS: Biochemistry of virus reproduction. Amer. J. Med. 38, 678 (1965).

TIMBURY. M. C.: The effect of anticellular serum on plaque formation by enteroviruses in human amnion tissue culture. Brit. J. exp. Path. 43, 506 (1962).

TIMBURY, M. C.: Antigenic variation in amnion cells after growth in tissue culture in relation to the inhibition of enteroviruses by anticellular serum. Virology 19, 501 (1963).

TOLBERT, O., B. WEAVER, and R. ENGLER: Synthesis of uncoated viral RNA during picornavirus infection. Arch. ges. Virusforsch. 19, 221 (1966).

TSILINSKY, Y. Y.: Inhibitors of viral activity from uninfected cultures of stable cell lines. I. Inhibition of the cytopathic effect, plaque formation and multiplication of some enteroviruses. Quantitative assay of the inhibitors. Acta virol. 7, 350 (1963a).

TSILINSKY, Y. Y.: Inhibitors of viral activity from uninfected cultures of stable cell lines. III. Interaction of inhibitors with trypsinized monkey kidney cells. Acta virol. 7, 542 (1963b).

TSILINSKY, Y. Y.: Inhibitors of viral activity from uninfected cultures of stable cell lines. II. Properties of inhibitors. Acta virol. 7, 436 (1963c).

TSILINSKY, Y. Y.: The ability of inhibitors of viral activity to slow down nonspecific degeneration of monkey kidney cell cultures. Acta virol. 7, 479 (1963d).

TSILINSKY, Y. Y., and V. S. LEVASHEV: Inhibitors of viral activity from uninfected cultures of stable cell lines. IV. Study of the relationship between the contamination of cell cultures with pleuropneumonia-like organisms (PPLO) and occurrence of inhibitors. Acta virol. 7, 549 (1963).

TYRRELL, D. A. J., and R. J. CHANOCK: Rhinoviruses: a description. Science 141, 152 (1963).

TYRRELL, D. A. J., S. K. R. CLARKE, R. B. HEATH, R. C. CURRAN, T. S. L. BESWICK, and L. WOLMAN: Studies of a coxsackievirus antigenically related to ECHO 9 virus and associated with an epidemic of aseptic meningitis with exanthem. Brit. J. exp. Path. 39, 178 (1958).

TYRRELL, D. A. J., and B. SNELL: Recovery of a virus from cases of an epidemic exanthem associated with meningitis. Lancet 271, 1028 (1956).

VASILENKO, S., and S. ATSEV: Experimental infection of mice with ECHO 6 virus. Acta virol. 9, 541 (1965).

VERLINDE, J. D., and J. B. WILTERDINK: Neuropathogenicity of non-polio enteroviruses with special reference to ECHO 9 virus. Folia psychiat. neerl. 61, 670 (1958).

VERLINDE, J. D., J. B. WILTERDINK, and R. P. MOUTON: Presence of two interfering enteroviral agents (ECHO virus type 9 and poliovirus type 2) in the human central nervous system. Arch. ges. Virusforsch. 10, 399 (1961).

WALLGREN, A.: Une nouvelle maladie infectieuse du système nerveux central. Acta paediat. (Uppsala) 4, 158 (1924).

WALLIS, C., A. M. BEHBEHANI, L. H. LEE, and M. BIANCHI: The infectiveness of organic iodine (Wescodyne) as a viral disinfectant. Amer. J. Hyg. 78, 325 (1963).

WALLIS, C., and J. L. MELNICK: Cationic stabilization — a new property of enteroviruses. Virology 16, 504 (1962).

WALLIS, C., and J. L. MELNICK: Irreversible photosensitization of viruses. Virology 23, 520 (1964).

WALLIS, C., and J. L. MELNICK: Differences in cystine dependence and chromatographic behavior between two type 4 ECHO virus strains. J. Bact. 89, 1310 (1965a).

WALLIS, C., and J. L. MELNICK: Photodynamic inactivation of enteroviruses. J. Bact. 89, 41 (1965b).

WALLIS, C., and L. J. MELNICK: Photodynamic inactivation of animal viruses: a review. Photochem. Photobiol. 4, 159 (1965c).

WALLIS, C., and J. L. MELNICK: Infectivity of type 4 ECHO virus-antibody complex. Virology 26, 175 (1965d).

WALLIS, C., J. L. MELNICK, and M. BIANCHI: Factors influencing enterovirus and reovirus growth and plaque formation. Tex. Rep. Biol. Med. 20, 693 (1962).

WALLIS, C., J. L. MELNICK, and F. RAPP: Different effects of $MgCl_2$ and $MgSO_4$ on the thermostability of viruses. Virology 26, 694 (1965).

WALLIS, C., F. MORALES, J. POWELL, and J. L. MELNICK: Plaque enhancement of enteroviruses by magnesium chloride, cysteine, and pancreatin. J. Bact. 91, 1932 (1966).

WALLIS, C., W. PARKS, N. SAKURADA, and J. L. MELNICK: A rapid plaque method using vertical tube cultures for titration of viruses and neutralizing antibodies. Bull. Wld Hlth Org. 33, 795 (1965).

WEHRLE, P. F., M. E. JUDGE, M. C. PARIZEAU, O. CARBONARO, M. MILLER, and S. ZINBERG: Disability associated with ECHO virus infections. N.Y. St. J. Med. 59, 3941 (1959).

WENNER, H. A.: Problems in working with enteroviruses. Ann. N.Y. Acad. Sci. 101, 343 (1962a).

WENNER, H. A.: The ECHO viruses. Ann. N.Y. Acad. Sci. 101, 398 (1962b).

WENNER, H. A., I. ARCHETTI, and G. R. DUBES: Antigenic variations among type 1 polioviruses. A study of 16 wild-type strains and 5 variants. Amer. J. Hyg. 70, 66 (1959).

WENNER, H. A., P. HARMON, A. M. BEHBEHANI, H. ROUHANDEH, and P. KAMITSUKA: The antigenic heterogeneity of type 30 ECHO viruses. Amer. J. Epidem. 85, 240 (1966).

WENNER, H. A., M. E. SOERGEL, P. S. KAMITSUKA, P. PERINE, T. D. Y. CHIN, and T. Y. LOU: The Caldwell group of enteric viruses. 1. Isolation and properties; serologic distinctions from existent prototype strains, and several other candidate enteric viruses. Amer. J. Hyg. 78, 247 (1963).

WIGAND, R., and A. B. SABIN: Properties of ECHO types 22, 23, and 24 viruses. Arch. ges. Virusforsch. 11, 224 (1961).

WIGAND, R., and A. B. SABIN: Properties of epidemic strains of ECHO type 9 virus and observations on the nature of human infection. Arch. ges. Virusforsch. 11, 685 (1962).

WILSEN, A. A. J., H. PEISACH, and W. H. HOWARTH: A closed epidemic of acute aseptic meningitis caused by ECHO virus type 4. S. Afr. med. J. 35, 330 (1961).

WILTERDINK, J. B., et al.: A case of paralytic disease caused by ECHO 9 virus. Ned. T. Geneesk. 109, 1524 (1965).

WINKELSTEIN, W., Jr., D. T. KARZON, A. L. BARRON, and N. S. HAYNER: Epidemiologic observations on an outbreak of aseptic meningitis due to ECHO virus type 6. Amer. J. publ. Hlth 47, 741 (1957).

YCEOGLU, A. M., S. BERKOVICH, and S. MINKOWITZ: Acute glomerulonephritis associated with ECHO virus type 9 infection. J. Pediat. **69,** 603 (1966).

YOHN, D. S., and W. McD. HAMMON: ECHO 4 viruses: improved methods and strain selection for identification and serodiagnosis. Proc. Soc. exp. Biol. (N.Y.) **105,** 55 (1960).

YOSHIOKA, I., and D. M. HORSTMANN: Viremia in infection due to ECHO virus type 9. New Engl. J. Med. **262,** 224 (1960).

YOW, M. D., J. L. MELNICK, R. J. BLATTNER, and L. E. RASMUSSEN: Enteroviruses in infantile diarrhea. Amer. J. Hyg. **77,** 283 (1963).

ZAFFIRO, P.: La reazione di emoagglutino-inhibizione nei virus ECHO (tipi 3, 7, 10, 11, 12, e 19). Boll. Ist. sieroter. milan. **38,** 435 (1959).

ZEIPEL, G. V., and A. SVEDMYR: A study of the association of ECHO viruses to aseptic meningitis. Arch. ges. Virusforsch. **7,** 355 (1957).

* Referred to in literature but abstract not available.

Reoviruses

By

Leon Rosen

Pacific Research Section
Laboratory of Infectious Diseases
National Institute of Allergy and Infectious Diseases
National Institutes of Health, U.S. Public Health Service
Honolulu, Hawaii, U.S.A.

Table of Contents

I. Introduction

Reoviruses are ether-resistant icosahedral viruses 60 to 75 mμ in diameter which contain ribonucleic acid. They have been recovered from man and lower animals and are ubiquitous in their geographic distribution. At present, the importance of these viruses as a cause of human or animal disease is still largely unknown. As a result of having a number of unusual characteristics, reoviruses have attracted the attention of many workers in the relatively short time since they were first recognized. For example, investigators interested in the molecular aspects of virology have been attracted by the unusual double-helical ribonucleic acid of high molecular weight which reoviruses possess, while those interested in epidemiology have been attracted by the occurrence of apparently identical viruses in both man and an unusually wide variety of lower animals. This compilation is based on information available to the author as of October 31, 1966.

II. History

The term "reovirus" was proposed in 1959 (SABIN, 1959) as a group name for a number of viruses then classified (SABIN, 1956; RAMOS-ALVAREZ and SABIN, 1958) as being identical with, or related to, ECHO type 10 virus. The latter agent was first designated (RAMOS-ALVAREZ and SABIN, 1956) as HE (human enteric) type 4 virus and then as an ECHO virus (Committee on the ECHO Viruses 1955) because it met the criteria *originally* established for the latter group, namely, 1) recovery from human feces by use of primate cell cultures, 2) lack of pathogenicity for the usual laboratory animals, and 3) lack of relationship to previously described virus groups. It was recognized from the first (RAMOS-ALVAREZ and SABIN, 1954), however, that the cytopathic effect in unstained cell cultures of the virus which became the prototype strain of ECHO type 10 was different than the "poliomyelitis virus type" now known to be characteristic of the other ECHO viruses and those Coxsackie viruses which produce cytopathic effects in cell cultures. The poliomyelitis viruses, the Coxsackie viruses, and the other ECHO viruses are now grouped in a family known as the picornaviruses (MELNICK et al., 1963).

ECHO type 10 and the related viruses which were subsequently discovered were removed from the ECHO group principally because it was learned, 1) that they were much larger than the latter viruses, and 2) that they produced cytoplasmic inclusions not seen with the other ECHO viruses (MALHERBE and HARWIN, 1957; DROUHET, 1958; SHAVER et al., 1958). The use of the letters "r" and "e" to form the word "reovirus" was intended to stress the association of these viruses with both the respiratory and enteric tracts respectively. It was recognized, of course, that this was not an exclusive characteristic of the group.

About the time that the term "reovirus" was proposed, it was found (ROSEN, 1960) that two viruses that had previously been isolated from *Macaca* monkeys and designated SV$_{12}$ and SV$_{59}$ (HULL et al., 1956) were identical with two reovirus serotypes (types 1 and 2, respectively) which had been isolated from man.

Later, it was discovered (STANLEY, 1961 a) that a virus originally isolated from man in suckling mice and described in 1953 (STANLEY et al., 1953) as hepato-encephalomyelitis virus was identical with the reovirus serotype that had been designated type 3. Finally, after the morphologic aspects of reovirus replication in cells had been studied by electron microscopy (TOURNIER and PLISSIER, 1960) it was recognized (BERNHARD and GRANBOULAN, 1962) that the cytoplasmic inclusions which had been seen in some specimens of mouse ascites tumor cells a number of years previously (SELBY et al., 1954) were identical with those produced by reoviruses.

III. Classification and Nomenclature

Animal viruses are now generally divided into those containing deoxyribonucleic acid (DNA) and those containing ribonucleic acid (RNA). The reoviruses are one of the four major groups of RNA viruses presently recognized and are usually distinguished from the three other groups, namely, the picornaviruses, the myxoviruses, and the arboviruses, by the criteria of size (in the case of the picornaviruses) and resistance to lipid solvents (in the case of myxoviruses and arboviruses).

The reovirus strains isolated from man and lower animals, with the exception of those from domestic chickens, can be classified (ROSEN, 1960, 1962) into three serotypes, designated types 1, 2, and 3. In so far as they have been tested, reoviruses of the same serotype from various animal species are indistinguishable from each other. Recently, 77 virus strains with many of the characteristics of reoviruses were isolated from domestic chickens and classified (KAWAMURA et al., 1965) into 5 serotypes designated, "Uchida", TS_{17}, CS_{108}, TS_{142}, and OS_{161}. The antigenic relationship of these viruses to reovirus types 1, 2, or 3 has not as yet been studied in detail, but it has been noted that they do not agglutinate human erythrocytes, a characteristic of all previously known reoviruses.

A large number of viruses which were isolated from monkeys and which fell into 2 serotypes, designated SV_4 (HULL et al., 1956) and SV_{28} (HULL et al., 1958), were at one time classified in "CPE group 3" (HULL et al., 1958) with other isolates from monkeys which had been placed in serotypes designated SV_{12} and SV_{59} (HULL et al., 1956). As noted above, the latter two serotypes were eventually found to be identical with reoviruses isolated from man. SV_4 and SV_{28} were known to be antigenically related to each other and were originally classified with SV_{12} and SV_{59} because all four serotypes produced similar cytopathic effects in unstained cell cultures. It was recognized, however, that SV_4 and SV_{28}, unlike SV_{12} and SV_{59}, did not agglutinate human erythrocytes but did agglutinate *Macaca* monkey erythrocytes (HULL et al., 1956; ROSEN, 1960). SV_4 virus was subsequently shown to be much smaller than the reoviruses and to have a number of the properties of the picornaviruses (SATTAR and ROZEE, 1965). Consequently, there is now no reason to consider SV_4 and SV_{28} as reoviruses.

There are viruses which share some characteristics with reoviruses and which eventually may be classified with them when additional data become available and a formal scheme of classification for viruses is agreed upon. Two viruses which affect plants are in this category. These are wound tumor virus (WTV), an agent discovered (BLACK, 1944) by feeding wild-caught leafhoppers from the United States on plants in the laboratory, and rice dwarf virus (RDV), the agent of a naturally occurring disease of rice plants in Japan. RDV is also transmitted by leafhoppers (insects which suck juices of plants). WTV and RDV are among the relatively few viruses which have been shown to replicate in both plants and animals (leafhoppers), and they resemble reoviruses in size and configuration of the virion (BILS and HALL, 1962; FUKUSHI et al., 1962; FUKUSHI and SHIKATA, 1963a), in having double-helical RNA (BLACK and MARKHAM, 1963; GOMATOS and TAMM, 1963b; TOMITA and RICH, 1964; MIURA et al., 1966; SATO et al., 1966), in resistance to ether (data available only on WTV) (STREISSLE and MARAMOROSCH, 1963a), and in replication in the cytoplasm and not the nucleus of cells (FUKUSHI et al., 1962; FUKUSHI and SHIKATA, 1963b; SHIKATA and MARAMOROSCH, 1965, 1966). In view of the similarities between WTV and RDV, it would not be surprising if some of the many other leafhopper-borne viruses affecting plants (MARAMOROSCH, 1963) were also found to have similar properties.

It has been reported that WTV is related antigenically to the reoviruses (STREISSLE and MARAMOROSCH, 1963b) but the data presented were not convincing. Conversely, the absence of such a relationship has also been reported (GOMATOS and TAMM, 1963b), but again the evidence was not conclusive. In the first instance, it was not demonstrated that the reactions observed were specific; in the second, it was not established beyond question that the WTV antiserum which failed to react with the reovirus antigens did indeed contain antibody against WTV.

Inoculation of monkey and mouse fibroblast cell cultures with WTV produced no cytopathic effects, nor were pathogenic effects seen in suckling mice or hamsters inoculated subcutaneously or intranasally (GOMATOS and TAMM, 1963b). Purified WTV also did not agglutinate human erythrocytes. No evidence of viral replication was obtained when reovirus strains of each of the three serotypes were inoculated into a species of leafhopper known to be capable of transmitting WTV (STREISSLE and ROSEN, unpublished).

Under experimental conditions, WTV multiplies in an unusually wide variety of plants and produces tumors in some (BLACK, 1965) but its plant hosts and pathogenicity in nature are unknown. Both WTV and RDV, like many other leafhopper-borne viruses, have been shown to be transmitted transovarially by infected female leafhoppers to a varying percentage of their progeny (BLACK, 1953, 1959). RDV and WTV are not transmitted through the sperm of infected male leafhoppers when the latter are mated with uninfected females. Perhaps, this is because these viruses are not found in the nucleus of cells.

Two groups of viruses, each consisting of multiple serotypes, which are usually classified (CASALS and CLARKE, 1965) as arboviruses, are also now known to show some resemblance to reoviruses. These are the viruses causing the disease of sheep known as bluetongue, and those causing the disease of equines known as African horse-sickness. Although considered arboviruses by some because of their multiplication in and transmission by blood-sucking insects (mainly species of *Culicoïdes*), unlike most arboviruses, they are resistant to ether (HOWELL, 1962; STUDDERT, 1965). One strain of bluetongue virus has been shown to have a diameter similar to that of reoviruses and also a similar naked capsid consisting of 92 capsomeres (STUDDERT et al., 1966). Another strain of bluetongue virus has been shown to contain RNA and to replicate in the cytoplasm of cells (LIVINGSTON and MOORE, 1962). A strain of African horse-sickness virus has also been shown to have a diameter similar to that of the reoviruses and a capsid consisting of 92 subunits (POLSON and DEEKS, 1963).

One more virus which resembles the reoviruses in some respects is that causing a disease of silkworm moth *(Bombyx mori)* larvae characterized by the formation of polyhedra in the cytoplasm of the midgut epithelium. This virus has been found to have RNA which shows base pairing and other characteristics which suggest that it, like the RNA of reoviruses, is a double-helical molecule of large molecular weight (HAYASHI and KAWASE, 1964, 1965).

Although there was speculation (MARAMOROSCH, 1964; STANLEY et al., 1964a; BELL, 1965) that a virus lysing blue-green algae (SAFFERMAN and MORRIS, 1963) might share some of the characteristics of reoviruses, it is now known that this virus contains DNA, rather than RNA, and possesses a tail (SCHNEIDER et al., 1964). Thus, it resembles most bacteriophages and there is no reason to consider it with the reoviruses.

IV. Properties of the Virion
1. Morphology

The structure of the virion of reovirus types 1, 2, and 3 has been studied extensively by electron microscopy using the negative staining technique (RHIM et al., 1961; GOMATOS et al., 1962; JORDAN and MAYOR, 1962; SMITH and MELNICK, 1962; VASQUEZ and TOURNIER, 1962, 1964; DALES et al., 1965; GROSE et al., 1965; LOH et al., 1965; MAYOR et al., 1965; MAYOR and JORDAN, 1965; THOMAS and DELAIN, 1965; MÜLLER et al., 1966). Although the measurements obtained from the various studies differed somewhat, the data suggest that these differences could be the result of the varying technical methods and were not necessarily an indication of real differences between types or between strains of the same type. The isolated virion was found to consist of an inner core and a capsid and to be roughly hexagonal in profile. In the various investigations its average diameter ranged from about 56 to 77 mμ. The core, also hexagonal in profile, had an average diameter ranging from 29 to 46 mμ. The capsid consisted of an electron-dense inner layer and an outer layer of capsomeres. No envelope and no filamentous forms have been described.

The structure of the outer layer of the capsid has been interpreted in two different ways. In one interpretation, it was suggested that the outer layer consists of 92 hollow columnar capsomeres arranged in the form of an icosahedron, 80 of the capsomeres being hexagonal in cross section and 12 being pentagonal (JORDAN and MAYOR, 1962; VASQUEZ and TOURNIER, 1962; MAYOR et al., 1965). In the other, it was suggested that the capsid contains 92 holes each surrounded by either 5 or 6 truncated pyramids arranged in icosahedral symmetry (VASQUEZ and TOURNIER, 1964). In this interpretation there would be 180 truncated pyramids each roughly triangular in cross section.

Less information is available on the morphology of the virions of the serotypes described from chickens. The average diameter of the virion of the 5 serotypes ranged from 70 to 82 mμ and the average diameter of the cores from 48 to 53 mμ. The shape of the entire virion, the core, and the detailed morphology of the capsid appeared similar to that described for reovirus types 1, 2, and 3 (KAWAMURA et al., 1965).

2. Chemical Composition

The chemical composition of reoviruses has been studied largely with strains of types 1 and 3. There is no evidence that significant differences exist among the reoviruses with respect to chemical composition and hence the data obtained with different serotypes will be considered together.

The virion is estimated to have a molecular weight of about 70 million daltons (molecular weight units) and apparently consists solely of protein and RNA (GOMATOS and TAMM, 1963a). The average buoyant density of purified whole virus preparations ranges from 1.36 to 1.38 gm/ml (GOMATOS and TAMM, 1963a; MAYOR et al., 1965; FOUAD and ENGLER, 1966). Reoviruses are resistant to the action of ethyl ether (SABIN, 1959; ROSEN et al., 1960a; KAWAMURA et al., 1965) and thus can be presumed to be devoid of peripheral structural lipids. Polysaccharides were not detected in reovirus inclusions when the latter were stained by the periodic acid — Schiff technique (DROUHET, 1960) and the absence of DNA in reoviruses is indicated by a negative reaction of the inclusions with the Feulgen stain (DROUHET, 1960; GOMATOS et al., 1962), a negative reaction of purified virus with diphenylamine (GOMATOS and TAMM, 1963a), and the lack of inhibition of replication by 5-fluro-2'-deoxyuridine (FUDR), 5-bromo-2'-deoxyuridine (BUDR), 5-iodo-2'-deoxyuridine (IUDR) and cytosine arabinoside (GOMATOS et al., 1962; KAWAMURA et al., 1965; SILAGI, 1965; LOH and SOERGEL, 1967).

The capsid of reoviruses can be removed by digestion with trypsin and pepsin and the latter enzyme also removes some material in the core of the virion, suggesting that it also contains some protein material (BERNHARD and TOURNIER, 1962; DALES et al., 1965; MAYOR et al., 1965). Ribonuclease and deoxyribonuclease have no effect on the capsid. Since the capsid appears to consist of two distinct layers which are not equally affected by various physical and chemical agents, the presence of more than one type of protein is implied (DALES et al., 1965).

The virion contains an unusually large amount of RNA (at least 10 million daltons) (GOMATOS and TAMM, 1963a; MAYOR et al., 1965) as compared with most RNA-containing viruses, and this RNA is further distinguished by the fact that it has a double-helical configuration. This unusual configuration for a virus RNA was originally suggested (GOMATOS et al., 1962) by the yellow-green staining of reovirus inclusion bodies by acridine orange — a reaction previously considered characteristic of DNA. The double-helical structure was confirmed by base composition analysis, thermal denaturation studies (GOMATOS and TAMM, 1963a, c), X-ray diffraction studies (LANGRIDGE and GOMATOS, 1963; ARNOTT et al., 1966), and the width of the RNA as visualized by electron microscopy (GOMATOS and STOECKENIUS, 1964; KLEINSCHMIDT et al., 1964).

It has not been possible to extract infectious RNA from purified reoviruses by techniques which have proven successful with picornaviruses (MAYOR et al., 1965). It is hypothesized that this is the result of the difficulty of extracting the double-helical reovirus RNA molecule(s) intact with currently available procedures (GOMATOS and STOECKENIUS, 1964; KLEINSCHMIDT et al., 1964; MAYOR et al., 1965).

3. Antigenic Composition

The reoviruses from both man and lower animals, with the exception of those isolated from chickens, can be grouped by hemagglutination-inhibition techniques in three serotypes which have been designated types 1, 2, and 3 (ROSEN, 1960). Neutralization techniques can also be used for typing (SABIN, 1959; BEHBEHANI et al., 1966) but are technically more difficult and often yield results less easy to interpret. Reovirus types 1, 2, and 3 share a common complement-fixing antigen (SABIN, 1959) but this property has not been investigated in detail. In so far as they have been studied, types 1, 2, or 3 from humans are indistinguishable by antigenic (or other) properties from strains isolated from lower animals (ROSEN, 1962). Human volunteers infected experimentally with a type 1 strain of bovine origin, and calves infected experimentally with each of the three serotypes of human origin, exhibited antigenic responses similar to those seen in natural infections (ROSEN and ABINANTI, 1960; KASEL et al., 1963). Moreover, the calves transmitted their infection to another calf in contact with them.

Hemagglutination-inhibition tests reveal antigenic relationships among all three types, but types 1 and 2 appear to be more closely related to each other than either is to type 3. Humans and lower animals infected with type 3 almost always show only a homotypic hemagglutination-inhibition antibody response whereas those infected with types 1 or 2 often develop hemagglutination-inhibition antibodies to the two heterotypic types (ROSEN et al., 1960a, b, 1963a, b). Strains of type 2 show the greatest antigenic variation. It has been suggested (HARTLEY et al., 1962) that subtypes can be recognized within this serotype but, since relatively few strains have been studied, it is uncertain that all strains will fall into discrete subtypes. A reovirus strain (from cattle) which has been proposed as a possible fourth serotype (MOSCOVICI et al., 1961) is probably a strain of type 2 (ROSEN, 1962).

Reoviruses isolated from chickens have been classified by neutralization tests in five serotypes designated "Uchida", TS_{17}, CS_{108}, TS_{142}, and OS_{161} (KAWAMURA et al., 1965). Antigenic relationships among these types have been demonstrated by neutralization, complement-fixation, and agar-gel diffusion tests and by fluorescent-antibody studies (KAWAMURA and TSUBAHARA, 1966). Antisera against the five chicken serotypes did not neutralize representative strains of types 1, 2, or 3 (KAWAMURA, personal communication).

4. Effects of Physical and Chemical Agents on Infectivity

Reoviruses are relatively resistant to inactivation by heat. One strain of type 1 was found to have a half-life at 4°, 24°, and 37° C of 3.7 days, 2.0 days, and 19 hours, respectively (RHIM et al., 1961). Another strain of type 1 dropped

2 log units in titer at 36.5° C in 3 weeks and the same amount in titer at 56° C in 30 minutes (HALONEN, 1961). A strain of type 3 was found to have a half-life at 37°, 45°, 56° C of 157, 33 and 1.6 minutes, respectively (GOMATOS et al., 1962).

Like enteroviruses, reoviruses are protected from loss of titer when heated for 1 hour at 50° C in the presence of M MgCl$_2$ (WALLIS and MELNICK, 1962; KAWAMURA et al., 1965). However, unlike enteroviruses, the infective titer of two strains of type 1 was *increased* by heating in the presence of high concentrations (0.25 M or more) of MgCl$_2$ (WALLIS et al., 1964). Other divalent cations did not have a similar effect. The infectivity of the same strains was decreased at *certain* subzero temperatures in the presence of high concentrations of MgCl$_2$ *and* other divalent cations (WALLIS et al., 1964). The mechanism of this altered response to temperature change is not known. It could not be attributed to dispersion of virus particles by heat nor their aggregation by cold.

Strains of reovirus type 1 were found to be susceptible to inactivation by visible light when photosensitized with the heterocyclic dyes, proflavine, neutral red, and toluidine blue (HIATT, 1960; WALLIS and MELNICK, 1964). Enteroviruses were not photosensitive under the same conditions. It is hypothesized that these dyes penetrate the protein coat of the virion and are bound to the nucleic acid.

The treatment of type 1 reovirus with proflavine in the absence of light results either in the diminution or the complete suppression of the cytopathic effect of the virus in cell cultures, depending on the concentration of dye employed (ZALAN and LABZOFFSKY, 1965). Furthermore, in cell cultures inoculated with virus exposed to certain concentrations of proflavine, no cytopathic effect is seen but the cells become resistant to infection with a wide variety of viruses including reoviruses. Exposure of the virus to higher concentrations of proflavine results in the inactivation of both cytopathic and interfering activity. It is not clear from the description of the above experiments whether or not the effect observed could have been influenced by visible light. Although it was stated that the actual treatment of virus with proflavine was carried out with the exclusion of light, no comment was made on whether or not measures were taken to prevent the possible effect of visible light during subsequent manipulations.

Strains of reovirus type 1, 2, and 3 were inactivated by ultraviolet light (RAUTH, 1965; McCLAIN and SPENDLOVE, 1966) but were more resistant to such inactivation than other RNA viruses which are known to possess single-stranded nucleic acid. Since reoviruses were similar in sensitivity to certain DNA viruses (which contain double-helical nucleic acid), it has been hypothesized that their relative resistance was due, at least in part, to the double-helical nature of their nucleic acid and that ultraviolet inactivation of viruses in general is independent of the form of sugar in their nucleic acid (RAUTH, 1965).

Certain anomalous effects were observed after exposure of reovirus types 1, 2, and 3 to ultraviolet light, or to reovirus types 1 and 2 sensitized with pro-flavine to visible light, which have been interpreted as evidence for the occurrence of "multiplicity reactivation" (McCLAIN and SPENDLOVE, 1966). The latter is defined as the production of virus by a cell infected by two or more damaged virus particles which individually are not capable of replicating.

Reovirus types 1 and 3 were not inactivated by exposure to a wide pH range

(STANLEY et al., 1953; KETLER et al., 1962). Similarly, the five chicken serotypes did not decrease in infectivity when exposed to a pH of 3.0 at 4° C for 24 hours (KAWAMURA et al., 1965). At low pH levels, reovirus type 1 was not activated at high temperatures nor inactivated at low temperatures in the presence of $MgCl_2$ as described above (WALLIS et al., 1964).

Infectivity titers of *some* preparations of reovirus types 1, 2, and 3 were increased by treatment with certain proteolytic enzymes (SPENDLOVE and SCHAFFER, 1965). This effect was not additive to that produced by heating in the presence of $MgCl_2$. It is hypothesized that the effect of both heating in $MgCl_2$ and of treatment with proteolytic enzymes is on potentially infectious particles which make up a large part of the untreated virus preparation.

A strain of type 1 (SV_{12}) was inactivated in less than 96 hours at 37° C by 1:4,000 formaldehyde (HULL et al., 1956) and a strain of type 2 (SV_{59}) was inactivated by the same concentration of formaldehyde at the end of 48 hours (HULL et al., 1958). The infectivity of reovirus types 1 and 2 was also reduced by the sulfhydryl reagents para-chloromercuribenzoate (PCMB) and iodoacetamide (ALLISON et al., 1962).

Reoviruses are relatively resistant to the commonly used germicidal agents. A strain of type 3 was resistant to the action of penicillin, streptomycin and chlortetracycline and survived exposure to 2% Lysol, 3% formaldehyde solution, 1% hydrogen peroxide or 1% phenol at room temperature for 1 hour. On the other hand, it was completely inactivated by 70% ethyl alcohol at room temperature for 1 hour or 3% formaldehyde at 56° C for 30 minutes (STANLEY et al., 1953, 1954).

V. Interaction with Cells in vitro

1. Host-cell Range and Assay of Infectivity

Reovirus types 1, 2, and 3 replicate and produce cytopathic effects in a remarkably wide variety of cell cultures. These include cultures derived from a variety of domestic animals as well as those of primate origin (HSIUNG, 1958; LENAHAN and WENNER, 1960). The cell culture which has been the most widely used for the recovery of these reoviruses from nature is primary *Macaca* (rhesus) monkey kidney. In addition, KB cells, HeLa cells, stable human amnion lines, primary human kidney, primary *Cercopithecus* kidney, BS-C-1 cells (*Cercopithecus* kidney line), and L cells (of murine origin), among others, have been used in a variety of studies including those on viral replication described below. There is evidence (McCLAIN et al., 1967) that various types of cells differ in their suitability for use in different types of experimental procedures but this point has not been investigated in detail. It should be noted that reovirus type 1 is often present in a "latent" state in primary cultures of both *Macaca* and *Cercopithecus* kidneys (HULL et al., 1956, 1958; HULL and MINNER, 1957; MALHERBE and HARWIN, 1957; MALHERBE et al., 1963), but this has not been recognized as a problem in most laboratory studies.

Strains of reovirus types 1, 2, and 3 produce satisfactory plaques on *Macaca* kidney (RHIM and MELNICK, 1961 a, b), BS-C-1 cells (McCLAIN et al., 1967), and L cells (FRANKLIN, 1961). Earlier difficulties in obtaining plaques with these viruses have been attributed to the inhibiting effect of the type of agar employed (WALLIS et al., 1962) and to neutral red and animal sera in the overlay medium (RHIM and MELNICK, 1961 b). Improved plaquing is obtained by incorporating pancreatin into the agar overlay (WALLIS et al., 1966). It has been shown (McCLAIN et al., 1967) that plaquing efficiency is influenced by virus strain, type of cell culture used in assay, and prior treatment of inocula with proteolytic enzymes.

In addition to plaque assay, an immunofluorescent cell count technique can also be used for infectivity assays of reovirus types 1, 2, and 3 (SPENDLOVE et al., 1963 b, 1964; McCLAIN et al., 1967). This technique has some advantages, such as speed and applicability to virus strains which do not form satisfactory plaques. It has the disadvantage that the cells and virus are killed in the course of the procedure and thus cannot be used as a source of viral clones.

Reoviruses isolated from chickens replicate and produce cytopathic effects in primary chicken kidney cell cultures (KAWAMURA et al., 1965) and plaques are also formed in this type of culture. None of the five chicken serotypes multiplied in swine kidney, guinea pig kidney, and bovine kidney or testis cell cultures (KAWAMURA, personal communication).

2. Reproductive Cycle

Reoviruses have a relatively prolonged reproductive cycle as compared with viruses containing single-stranded RNA and, unlike the latter, tend to remain cell-associated. Since the reproductive cycle of reoviruses is similar in duration to that of DNA viruses, it has been suggested that the relative length of the cycles of both types of viruses is a function of the double-helical nucleic acid which they possess. Reproductive cycles of types 1, 2, and 3 have been studied in several different cell culture systems (RHIM et al., 1961; GOMATOS et al., 1962; SPENDLOVE et al., 1963 b; OIE et al., 1966) and the results can be summarized as follows. Approximately 60—90% of the virus was adsorbed to cells at 37° C within two hours (if the amount adsorbed at four hours is considered equivalent to 100%). The latent period ranged from 6 to 9 hours and the maximum yields were obtained between 15 and 54 hours. At the time of maximum yield, only 7 to 53% of virus was extracellular. The total yield of virus ranged from 225 to 2600 plaque-forming units per cell. Although differences in reproductive characteristics were noted among the various serotypes, and between strains of the same serotype in different cell culture systems, it is not clear if these differences were in fact a function of these, or other, factors.

One study (SPENDLOVE et al., 1966) of a reovirus reproductive cycle utilized the discovery that the titers of some reovirus preparations can be enhanced by treatment with proteolytic enzymes (SPENDLOVE and SCHAFFER, 1965). In this study, yields were characterized as enzymatically enhanceable virus (PIV) or infectious virus (IV), i.e. virus detectable before enzyme treatment. It was found that the latent period was shorter, the rate of synthesis more rapid, and the total yield more than 10-fold greater, when PIV was compared with IV. It also appeared that PIV was selectively released, and IV selectively retained by cells, or alternatively, that the latter type of virus was more rapidly inactivated by heat.

3. Morphologic Aspects of Replication

a) Conventional Microscopy

The typical cytopathic effect of reovirus types 1, 2, and 3 in living unstained cell cultures is difficult to describe but usually can be recognized with experience, at least in *Macaca* kidney cells. It is different from that produced by most picornaviruses. Cells infected with reoviruses become granular and do not slough off glass as readily as do cells infected with picornaviruses. Often, they remain fastened to the glass by a single process and flutter in the medium as the tube is moved during microscopic examination. The typical cytopathic effect is often confused with non-specific cellular degeneration by inexperienced personnel. When relatively small amounts of virus are inoculated, a typical cytopathic effect sometimes is not seen before the cells actually do degenerate nonspecifically. It is reported that the cytopathic effects of these types appear sooner when infected cell cultures are incubated on a roller drum (LERNER et al., 1962a) but this has not been a consistent finding (ROSEN, unpublished; RHIM et al., 1965). Chicken kidney cell cultures infected with reoviruses from chickens first show vacuolization of infected cells and then form syncytia (KAWAMURA et al., 1965).

In conventional microscopy of stained cells of many types infected with reovirus types 1, 2, and 3, single or multiple cytoplasmic inclusions of varying sizes and forms, which stain red with hematoxylin and eosin and blue with Giemsa, are seen in the perinuclear area (MALHERBE and HARWIN, 1957; DROUHET, 1958; SHAVER et al., 1958; SABIN, 1959; LA PLACA, 1962; RHIM et al., 1962; MALHERBE et al., 1963). These are first seen about 6 hours after inoculation and later appear to coalesce and fill the cytoplasm almost entirely, often forming a partial or complete ring around the nucleus. No specific lesions have been described in the nucleus. In cells infected with chicken reoviruses, small cytoplasmic inclusions which stain with *both* hematoxylin and eosin are seen 10 hours after inoculation. Later, they enlarge, appear more basophilic, and are seen around the congregated nuclei of syncytia (KAWAMURA et al., 1965).

The location of viral antigen within cells infected with reovirus types 1, 2, and 3 has been studied extensively by the use of fluorescent antibody (DROUHET, 1960; GOMATOS et al., 1962; RHIM et al., 1962; SPENDLOVE et al., 1963a, b, 1964; JONCAS, 1964; OIE et al., 1966). Viral antigen can be detected in particulate form in the cytoplasm as early as 4 hours post-inoculation, but usually appears several hours later. The particles coalesce to form a reticulum-like structure throughout the cytoplasm and, eventually, this reticulum is concentrated in the perinuclear area. Thus, the viral antigen is seen to occupy the same part of the cytoplasm as the inclusions seen by conventional staining. Viral antigen was not detected in the nucleus. In the course of one of these studies, it was noted (SPENDLOVE et al., 1963a) that viral antigen was localized in the areas occupied by the spindles and centrioles in *dividing cells* and that such antigen was transferred to daughter cells. In cells infected in the presence of spindle poisons, viral antigen developed in normal amounts but formed spherical globules rather than a reticulum. Antimitotic agents which do not disrupt the mitotic spindle had no effect on the arrangement of viral antigen (SPENDLOVE et al., 1964).

Cytochemical studies employing acridine orange have also been carried out with cells infected with reovirus types 1, 2, and 3 (GOMATOS et al., 1962; RHIM et al., 1962; MAYOR, 1965; OIE et al., 1966). It was found that the cytoplasmic inclusions usually stain yellow-green, a reaction now believed to be indicative of the presence of double-helical nucleic acid. This staining is not prevented by prior treatment of the cells with deoxyribonuclease or ribonuclease. In some types of cell cultures, the inclusions and the cytoplasmic area around them stain red in the later stages of the reproductive cycle. The red staining is prevented by prior treatment of the cells with ribonuclease but not by deoxyribonuclease. When the red staining is prevented by ribonuclease, the inclusions stain green. No indications of the presence of viral nucleic acid were seen in the nucleus. The above staining reactions have been interpreted (MAYOR, 1965) as indicative of the presence of double-helical viral RNA (the type found in the mature virion) in the inclusions throughout the reproductive cycle accompanied by the appearance of a single-stranded RNA of unknown function in the cytoplasm late in the cycle.

b) Electron Microscopy

The morphologic aspects of the replication of reovirus types 1, 2, and 3 have also been studied extensively by electron microscopy of ultrathin sections of infected cells (TOURNIER and PLISSIER, 1960; HARFORD et al., 1962; LA PLACA, 1962; RHIM et al., 1962; DALES, 1963; DALES et al., 1965; MAYOR and JORDAN, 1965; THOMAS and DELAIN, 1966a, b). It appears that the virion is taken into the cell with its capsid intact. In one of these studies (DALES et al., 1965), in which autoradiography was also employed, virions were seen singly within vacuoles and in aggregations in larger inclusions within 2 hours after inoculation. Evidence of digestion of the capsid in these inclusions was seen in cells 4 hours after inoculation. The intracellular release of labelled viral RNA from the inoculum was highly asynchronous and it was not possible to trace the transfer of RNA from the inclusions to the site of viral replication. Thus, there was no direct evidence that the virions in the inclusions were the source of parental RNA. However, the absence of intact virions, viral nucleoids, or labelled RNA in other areas of the cytoplasm during the first few hours after inoculation suggested that the parental RNA does come from this source. The later appearance of labelled material at the sites of replication indicated that some inoculum RNA passes to that region.

Vesicles form in infected cells in certain areas of the cytoplasm, mainly in the perinuclear region, before the appearance of progeny virus (MAYOR and JORDAN, 1965). Later in the reproductive cycle, aggregates of virus particles are seen in juxtaposition to, but not in, these vesicular regions. The virus matrices apparently coalesce as the cycle progresses and sometime contain numerous viral particles packed in "crystalline" arrays. These matrices correspond in size and position to the inclusions seen by conventional microscopy. Both complete virions, 60 to 75 mμ in diameter with an electron-dense central core, *and* empty capsids are seen in the matrices. The matrices also contain long hollow structures which have been identified (DALES, 1963) as the spindle tubules of the mitotic apparatus. In some instances, these tubules are partially or completely surrounded by a coat of electron-dense material and virus particles are seen to be next to, or embedded in, this coating substance. Studies with ferritin-conjugated antibody suggest that the coating substance is antigenically related to reovirus protein (DALES et al., 1965). Treatment of cells with colchicine (a spindle poison) results in the disappearance of the spindle tubules without affecting viral replication. Specific changes were not detected in the nucleus by electron microscopy, but a small amount of radioactive tracer material was detected there by autoradiography (DALES et al., 1965). The significance of the latter finding is unknown.

4. Chemical Aspects of Replication

In L cells infected with reovirus type 3 or human amnion cells infected with reovirus type 2, there is no inhibition of cellular DNA, RNA, or protein synthesis until the time that progeny virus begins to form (about 8 hours after inoculation). After that time, there is marked inhibition of DNA synthesis, some inhibition of protein synthesis, but no detectable inhibition of RNA synthesis (GOMATOS and TAMM, 1963d; KUDO and GRAHAM, 1965; LOH and SOERGEL, 1967).

Replication of reovirus type 3 in the L cell culture system is only temporarily suppressed by exposure of the cells to streptovitacin A for two hours after virus inoculation (DALES, 1965). This suggests that it is not necessary for the host cell to synthesize protein at the time of inoculation in order to release RNA from the virion, but rather, that the necessary lytic enzymes are already in the cell prior to inoculation.

RNA synthesis of normal cells can be largely inhibited by a dosage of actinomycin D which does not affect reovirus replication (KUDO and GRAHAM, 1965; SHATKIN, 1965a; LOH and SOERGEL, 1966) — although larger dosages do so (GOMATOS et al., 1962). Using appropriate dosages of actinomycin D, it has been shown (KUDO and GRAHAM, 1965; SHATKIN and RADA, 1967) that with reovirus type 3 two types of virus-specific RNA are formed in infected cells beginning about 6 hours after inoculation. One type is double-helical and ribonuclease-resistant and thus resembles that in the mature virion. The other, which is present in larger amounts, is single-stranded, ribonuclease-sensitive, and may function as the virus messenger RNA (PREVEC and GRAHAM, 1966; SHATKIN and RADA, 1967). As noted above, both types of RNA also have been observed in viral inclusions by staining with acridine orange (MAYOR, 1965), but in that study the single-stranded form was seen only late in the reproductive cycle. Production of both types of RNA requires protein synthesis 6 to 9 hours after inoculation and there is evidence to suggest that the two types are synthesized by different enzymes (KUDO and GRAHAM, 1966; SHATKIN and RADA, 1967).

Although it was reported (GOMATOS et al., 1964, 1965; KRUG et al., 1965) that reovirus RNA can serve as a template for both RNA and DNA polymerases from *Escherichia coli*, it was subsequently shown (SHATKIN, 1965b) that this finding was probably the result of the contamination of the reovirus RNA with host cell DNA.

In addition to actinomycin D, replication of reovirus type 3 is inhibited to a greater or lesser degree by mitomycin C, 5,6-dibromo-1-β-D-ribofuranosyl-

benzimidazole, tubericidin, and 4-aminopteroylglutamic acid (aminopterin)
(GOMATOS et al., 1962; ACS et al., 1964). With a strain of reovirus type 2, a relatively high dose of actinomycin D inhibited the synthesis of viral RNA but
most of the infected cells continued to produce viral antigen (LOH and SOER-
GEL, 1965). The multiplication of all 3 reovirus serotypes was insensitive to
the inhibitory action of 2-(α-hydroxybenzyl)-benzimidazole (HBB) (EGGERS
and TAMM, 1961), and the multiplication of type 1 was insensitive to inhibition
by guanidine (RIGHTSEL et al., 1961).

5. Hemagglutination

A strain of simian origin (SV_{12}) was the first reovirus reported (HULL et al.,
1956) to hemagglutinate and, as far as is known, all strains of reovirus types 1,
2, and 3 possess the property of agglutinating human erythrocytes. It is generally
more difficult to demonstrate agglutination of human erythrocytes (and to
obtain high-titered hemagglutinins) for strains of type 3, than for strains of types 1
and 2 (ROSEN, 1960). Titers obtained with group A or AB erythrocytes are slightly
higher on the average for all three serotypes than those obtained with group B
or O (BRUBAKER et al., 1964). Reoviruses of all three serotypes agglutinate
human erythrocytes to the same titer at 4°, 23°, and 37° C and no effect of pH
is seen in the range from 6.0 to 8.0 (HALONEN, 1961). Strains of type 3, but
not those of types 1 and 2, also agglutinate bovine erythrocytes at 4° C (EGGERS
et al., 1962). With a strain of reovirus type 3 and bovine erythrocytes, it was
found that one hemagglutinating unit corresponds to 6.2×10^6 plaque-forming
units (GOMATOS and TAMM, 1962). However, since coreless capsids, as well as
complete virions, apparently can hemagglutinate (FOUAD and ENGLER, 1966),
it is obvious that the quantitative relationship between hemagglutination and
infectivity will vary depending on the proportion of the former type of particles
in the preparation tested. Reovirus hemagglutinins can be prepared in a variety
of cell cultures including both cell lines and cell strains (RHIM et al., 1965).
It has been reported (LERNER et al., 1962a) that higher hemagglutinin
titers are obtained in rolled cultures, but others (ROSEN, unpublished; RHIM
et al., 1965) have obtained equal or better results with stationary cultures. Reovirus hemagglutinins are comparatively stable at temperatures ranging from
4° to 37° C but are rapidly inactivated at 56° C (HALONEN, 1961; USMANKHOD-
ZHAYEV and ZAKSTELSKAYA, 1964). Differences in thermostability were noted
among types 1, 2, and 3, but, since only a single strain of each type was examined,
it is not clear if the differences observed are characteristic of the various serotypes
or merely of the particular strains employed. The reoviruses isolated from chickens
do not agglutinate human or chicken erythrocytes at either 4° or 37° C (KAWAMURA
et al., 1965).

Treatment of human erythrocytes with *Vibrio cholerae* filtrate (RDE) has
no effect on their susceptibility to agglutination by reovirus types 1, 2, and 3
(GOLDFIELD et al., 1957; SABIN, 1959; LERNER et al., 1963). RDE does render
bovine erythrocytes inagglutinable by reovirus type 3 (GOMATOS and TAMM,
1962). However, two strains with differing properties in this respect were obtained
from a single isolate of reovirus type 3 (NEWLIN and McKEE, 1966). One of the
strains agglutinates only human erythrocytes, the other both human and bovine

erythrocytes. The erythrocyte receptors for the strain which agglutinates only human erythrocytes are not affected by RDE, whereas the receptors on *both* human and bovine erythrocytes for the other strain are affected.

A great variety of both known chemical compounds and complex substances of biologic origin have been tested for their effect on either the hemagglutinating ability of reoviruses or the susceptibility of erythrocytes to agglutination by these viruses (DARDANONI and ZAFFIRO, 1958; BUCKLAND, 1959, 1960; GOMATOS and TAMM, 1962; HALONEN and PYHTILA, 1962; ZALAN et al., 1962b; BUCKLAND and TYRRELL, 1963; LERNER et al., 1963, 1965, 1966a, b; SCHMIDT et al., 1964a, b, c; USMANKHODZHAYEV and ZAKSTELSKAYA, 1964; WALLIS et al., 1964; GELB and LERNER, 1965; ROSSER et al., 1965; SPENDLOVE and SCHAFFER, 1965; BENO and EDWARDS, 1966). Some of these materials increase hemagglutinin titers of virus preparations, some have no effect, and others decrease hemagglutinin titers. Contradictory results are sometimes reported by different laboratories (e.g. concerning the effect of proteolytic enzymes on virus preparations). Interpretation of the data is difficult since the purity of virus preparations employed and the conditions of treatment and testing varied considerably. Some of the tests have demonstrated differences between the hemagglutinating properties and erythrocyte receptors of reoviruses on the one hand and those of other hemagglutinating viruses on the other. However, as yet, it does not appear possible to interpret the data in a way which contributes to an understanding of the nature of reoviruses themselves, the mechanism of reovirus hemagglutination, or the reactions between reoviruses and cells in general.

VI. Interaction with Organisms

1. Host Range

Reoviruses have an exceptionally wide host range. Aside from man, reoviruses have been recovered from naturally infected wild and laboratory mice (types 2 and 3, respectively), dogs (type 1), cattle (types 1, 2, and 3), quokkas (short-tailed wallabies, a marsupial [type 3]), *Macaca* monkeys (types 1 and 2), *Cercopithecus* monkeys (type 1), chimpanzees (type 2), and chickens (5 chicken serotypes) (HULL et al., 1956; SABIN, 1960; HARTLEY et al., 1961; COOK, 1963; LOU and WENNER, 1963; MALHERBE et al., 1963; ROSEN et al., 1963a; STANLEY et al., 1964a; KAWAMURA et al., 1965; MASSIE and SHAW, 1966).

It is also reported that reoviruses were isolated from blood of seven species of wild birds and from pools of two species of culicine mosquitoes in New Zealand (MILES et al., 1965) and from pools of two other species of culicine mosquitoes in Western Australia (L. PARKER et al., 1965). All of these isolations were made in suckling mice. Both of the isolates from Australia and four of nineteen isolates from New Zealand (the only ones tested) were identified as type 3. The authors of both reports were aware of the occurrence of reoviruses in laboratory mouse colonies and the attempted re-isolations (in suckling mice) from the original material were successful in most instances. However, so few details are given in the original publications and the findings are of such potential importance, that, in view of the common occurrence of reovirus type 3 in mouse colonies (HARTLEY et al., 1961; ROWE et al., 1962; COOK, 1963), it cannot be considered as established that the isolates were indeed derived from the sources stated. Some of the mosquitoes in each of the positive pools from Australia were known to have been engorged, and hence it is possible that the isolates, if valid, were derived from recently ingested blood. No information was given on the presence or absence of engorged specimens in the ten positive mosquito pools from New Zealand.

Hemagglutination-inhibition or neutralizing "antibodies" against reovirus types 1, 2, or 3 have been reported in uninoculated trout, chickens, guinea pigs, rabbits, cats, dogs, swine, sheep, bats, wallabies, kangaroos, quokkas and several genera of New World monkeys (ROSEN, 1962; STANLEY and LEAK, 1963; STANLEY et al., 1964a). It is not known if such "antibodies" reflect actual previous infection with these reoviruses, but it seems likely that most of those observed in mammals and marsupials do.

The species of animals which have been infected experimentally with reovirus types 1, 2, or 3 are mice (STANLEY et al., 1953 and many others — see below), rats (STANLEY et al., 1953), hamsters (THOMAS et al., 1965), guinea pigs (ROSEN, 1960), dogs (LOU and WENNER, 1963; MASSIE and SHAW, 1966; HOLZINGER and GRIESEMER, 1966), *Macaca* monkeys (STANLEY et al., 1954; HULL et al., 1956, 1958; WENNER and CHIN, 1957), chimpanzees (SABIN, 1960) and cattle (ROSEN and ABINANTI, 1960; LAMONT, 1966; TRAINOR et al., 1966). The data with respect to ferrets and rabbits are equivocal (LOU and WENNER, 1963), although the latter species develops high antibody titers following a single intravenous inoculation of virus.

No evidence of viral multiplication or long-term persistence was found in *Aedes aegypti* mosquitoes fed on suckling mice with reovirus type 3 viremia or directly on reovirus type 3 suspensions (SIMPSON et al., 1965). Virus persisted for a number of days, but no evidence of multiplication was found, in *Aedes australis* mosquitoes and *Erythroneura zealandica* leafhoppers inoculated intrathoracically with an unspecified type of reovirus (MILES et al., 1965). Reovirus types 1, 2, and 3 of human origin persisted for less than seven days in inoculated *Agallia constricta* leafhoppers (STREISSLE and ROSEN, unpublished).

2. Pathology and Pathogenesis in Lower Animals

a) Mice

Spontaneous disease caused by reovirus type 3 has been observed in mice in laboratory colonies (NELSON and COLLINS, 1961; COOK, 1963) and extensive virologic, histologic, and cytologic studies of experimental infections with reovirus types 1, 2, and 3 have been carried out in the same species (STANLEY et al., 1953, 1954, 1964b, 1966; VAN TONGEREN, 1957; WALTERS et al., 1963, 1965; NELSON, 1964; HASSAN et al., 1965; HOBBS and MASCOLI, 1965; JENSON et al., 1965; PAPADIMITRIOU, 1965, 1966; HASHIMI et al., 1966; HASSAN and COCHRAN, 1966; JOSKE et al., 1966; KUNDIN et al., 1966; KLEIN, 1967).

Spontaneous disease has been observed primarily in suckling mice. The signs observed included diarrhea, oily hair (probably due to an excess of fat in the feces), retardation of growth, and jaundice. At autopsy, the mice had yellow necrotic areas in the liver and enlarged protruding gall bladders. Jaundice and necrotic areas in the liver were also observed in some adult mice in contact with affected sucklings.

Suckling mice experimentally infected with a reovirus type 3 strain originally isolated in mice (STANLEY et al., 1953, 1954, 1964b; WALTERS et al., 1963; JOSKE et al., 1966) showed jaundice, steatorrhea, oily hair, retardation of growth, emaciation, signs of central nervous system disease, and in later stages, alopecia. The signs were at their height between 8 and 15 days after inoculation and, while a majority of the animals died, some survived and continued to show signs of disease for many months. At autopsy, the liver was enlarged and showed small circular yellow lesions. A bile-stained or hemorrhagic peritoneal exudate was frequently present and some animals had small gray lesions on the heart and hemorrhagic lesions in the lungs. Microscopically, the principal lesions were in the liver, central nervous system, and the pancreas. Lesser lesions were observed in salivary glands, the heart, lungs, and skeletal muscle. The pathologic picture was one of focal parenchymal degeneration and necrosis associated with mild inflammation. Splenic atrophy was observed in about one-half the mice which survived for more than one year. Microscopically, follicular atrophy and fibrosis were seen in the atrophic spleens.

In one laboratory (WALTERS et al., 1965), suckling mice infected with strains of reovirus types 1 and 2 reacted similarly to those infected with the type 3 strain except that a lower percentage of mice showed clinical evidence of infection. Gross lesions in the liver and heart were similar to those seen in type 3 infections, but less frequent. Microscopically, cardiac and pulmonary lesions were more, and central nervous system lesions less, prominent. Necrosis of brown fat was observed in type 1 infections — a finding also reported in experimental murine infections with an unknown type of reovirus (VAN TONGEREN, 1957). After several serial passages in suckling mice, both the type 1 and the type 2 strains produced a more severe disease in suckling mice. In another laboratory (HASSAN et al., 1965; JENSON et al., 1965) all suckling mice inoculated with a different strain of type 1 died 5 to 12 days after inoculation of myocarditis or encephalitis. Because of differences in strains, passage history, routes of inoculation and dosages, it is not known if the differences observed within and among the serotypes with respect to severity and character of clinical manifestations were characteristic of the particular strains or serotypes, or, were the result of other variables.

Electron microscopy has been used to study the brain (JENSON et al., 1965) and heart (HASSAN et al., 1965) of suckling mice infected with reovirus type 1 and the liver (PAPADIMITRIOU, 1965) of mice infected with type 3. In all three studies aggregates of virus particles, similar to those seen in infected cells *in vitro*, were seen in the cytoplasm of affected cells. The viral particles were sometimes in "crystalline" arrays and, again as in cells *in vitro*, both complete virions and empty capsids were seen. Cytoplasmic inclusions, also similar to those seen *in vitro*, were noted by conventional microscopy in the studies of the brain and heart.

In one study of suckling mice experimentally infected with reovirus type 3, virus titers reached their peak in the liver on the fourth day after infection and in the brain on the eighth or ninth day (STANLEY et al., 1953). This virus could also be isolated from the feces and from blood of mice early in the course of experimental infection (STANLEY et al., 1954) and from the brain as late as 70 days afterwards (STANLEY et al., 1964 b). In experimental infections with type 1, virus could be isolated from the blood at an early stage of infection but reached its peak in the heart and brain at 3 and 6 days, respectively (HASSAN et al., 1965; JENSON et al., 1965). In long-term experimental infections with types 1 and 2, virus was recovered from the brain at 42 and 35 days after infection, respectively (WALTERS et al., 1965). For all three serotypes, specific hemagglutination-inhibition antibody was observed in almost every experimental animal tested at an appropriate time in the course of infection.

Evidence in favor of the specificity of reovirus hemagglutination-inhibition antibody in mice (especially with respect to type 3) has been provided by the demonstration of the simultaneous but transitory appearance of complement-fixing antibody in a series of animals followed for a number of months (PARKER et al., 1966) and the absence of reovirus hemagglutination-inhibition antibody in germfree mice (J. C. PARKER et al., 1965).

Although *weanling* mice usually show no signs of infection following oral, intraperitoneal, intracerebral, or subcutaneous routes of inoculation with reoviruses (STANLEY et al., 1953; NELSON, 1964; KLEIN, 1967), clinical respiratory disease and death in weanling mice has been described (HOBBS and MASCOLI, 1965) following intranasal inoculation under ether anesthesia of reovirus types 1, 2, and 3. Since adequate controls were not employed, it is not clear if the pathology observed was due to reovirus infection alone or to an aspiration pneumonia, or to both. Virus was recovered both from the lungs of mice which became sick and from those of mice which remained well. In other experiments (NELSON, 1964), reovirus type 3 was recovered from liver, brain, blood, intestinal washings and peritoneal washings of weanling mice one week after inoculation, and from peritoneal washings as long as 18 weeks afterwards.

Extensive virologic, serologic, and histologic studies have been carried out (HASHIMI et al., 1966) on mice born of mothers inoculated intraperitoneally at various times during gestation with reovirus type 2. The data are difficult to interpret since it is not known when the observed mice became infected. Although the authors assumed that all mice became infected *in utero* at the time that their mothers were inoculated, it is also possible that at least some mice became infected at a later time — even postpartum. About one-fourth of the mice became ill within two weeks of birth and one-half of the total number in the next three weeks. Homotypic hemagglutination-inhibition antibody was found in most mice tested at three weeks postpartum, but not in ten apparently well mice tested at three months of age. It was concluded that antibody observed in the younger mice was passively acquired maternal antibody and that the absence of antibody in the older animals indicated the establishment of tolerant infection with immune paralysis. However, this conclusion cannot be accepted without further evidence since it was not shown that the ten negative mice had been infected. Apparently, no attempt was made to isolate virus from these animals and no information was given on whether or not they had been ill at any time prior to the time that they were killed. It is possible that they were well *because* they had escaped infection.

In another study (HASSAN and COCHRAN, 1966), pregnant mice were inoculated with reovirus type 1 at various times during pregnancy and their uteri examined at 18 days of gestation for the presence of resorption sites and abnormal fetuses. It was found that there was a higher prevalence of fetal resorption, fetal death, and gross malformation in these mice as compared with mice inoculated with a poliomyelitis virus or control cell culture fluid.

Reoviruses have been recovered from a variety of ascites tumors and leukemias which were being passed in mice (BENNETTE, 1960; NELSON and TARNOWSKI, 1960; HARTLEY et al., 1961; THOMAS et al., 1965) but, with the one exception discussed below, it has not been suggested that reoviruses are etiologic agents of neoplasms in these animals. In fact, in two instances (BENNETTE, 1960; NELSON and TARNKOWSKI, 1960), reoviruses were detected because they sometimes destroyed the ascites tumors with which they were associated, and reoviruses have been used in laboratory experiments to render mice resistant to such tumors (KLEIN, 1967). In all instances where typing has been attempted, reoviruses isolated from neoplasms in laboratory mice have been identified as type 3.

In one instance (STANLEY et al., 1966), a lymphatous neoplasm was produced in suckling mice by the passage of spleen *cells* from a mouse inoculated 9 months previously with reovirus type 3. This tumor could be reproduced by further intraperitoneal passage of intact cells to suckling and adult mice (KEAST and STANLEY, 1966). Electron microscopy (PAPADIMITRIOU, 1966) failed to reveal the presence of reovirus-like particles in the tumor cells and no virus could be demonstrated in tests for infectivity (KEAST and STANLEY, 1966). It is reported that this mouse tumor shows a close relationship to Burkitt's lymphoma of man (see below) with respect to its anatomical distribution, its appearance by conventional and electron microscopy, and the properties of its cells in culture (JOSKE et al., 1966). It has been hypothesized (STANLEY and WALTERS, 1966) that the tumor was caused by reovirus type 3 but that the tumor cells contain only the non-infectious genome of this virus. The evidence advanced (STANLEY, 1966b) for the latter point is that the tumor cells contain an antigen which reacts as a specific reovirus type 3 antigen in complement-fixation tests. Data to substantiate the specificity of the reaction, and to demonstrate the absence of complete virus from tumor cell antigen, have not as yet been published.

b) Primates Other Than Man

An outbreak of upper respiratory disease apparently caused by reovirus type 2 was observed among chimpanzees housed in a laboratory (SABIN, 1960). The same syndrome was reproduced by nasal instillation of cell-culture-grown virus into chimpanzees without antibody. In these animals, virus was recovered from nasal secretions and, in greater concentration, from the feces for as long as two weeks. Both the naturally and the experimentally infected animals developed antibody. Reovirus type 2 has also been recovered from the lung of a *Macaca* monkey which died with an interstitial pneumonitis acquired in captivity (N. G. ROGERS, personal communication; HULL et al., 1956).

Hepatitis was observed in a *Macaca* monkey experimentally infected by the oral route with reovirus type 3 (STANLEY et al., 1954), and neuronal de-

generation, meningitis, and necrosis of the choroid plexus was seen in the same
genus inoculated intracerebrally or intramuscularly with types 1 and 2 (HULL
et al., 1956, 1958; WENNER and CHIN, 1957). Reoviruses have been recovered
from the feces of *Macaca* (HULL et al., 1958) and *Cercopithecus* (MALHERBE
et al., 1963) monkeys held in captivity and also from the mouth of the latter
genus. Reovirus types 1 and 3 have also been recovered from the blood of experimentally infected *Macaca* monkeys (STANLEY et al., 1954; LOU and WENNER,
1963).

Reovirus type 1 is commonly isolated from uninoculated cultures of cells
from the kidneys of *Macaca* (HULL and MINNER, 1957) and *Cercopithecus* (MAL-
HERBE et al., 1963) monkeys under conditions which suggest that, at least in
some instances, the viruses originated in the cells themselves and were not
introduced into the cultures from other sources.

c) Cattle

Naturally acquired disease caused by reoviruses has not been reported in
cattle, but a mild respiratory illness has been produced in calves experimentally
inoculated with a strain of reovirus type 1 of human origin (TRAINOR et al.,
1966). In other experiments (LAMONT, 1966), no clinical signs were seen following
experimental infection of calves with a bovine strain of reovirus type 1 but
macroscopic and microscopic signs of interstitial pneumonia were found when
the animals were killed.

Reoviruses of all three types may be detected in the feces of naturally and
experimentally infected cattle (ROSEN and ABINANTI, 1960; MOSCOVICI et al.,
1961; ROSEN et al., 1963a) for as long as one month, although they are usually
present for shorter periods of time. Reoviruses have also been recovered from
nasal and conjunctival swabs of experimentally infected animals, as well as
from their blood, lungs, and lymph nodes (ROSEN and ABINANTI, 1960; LAMONT,
1966; TRAINOR et al., 1966). Both naturally and experimentally infected cattle
regularly develop homologous (and sometimes heterologous) hemagglutination-
inhibition antibody. Passively acquired maternal antibody does not appear to
protect cattle from infection under natural conditions (ROSEN et al., 1963a).

d) Dogs

Reovirus type 1 was recovered from the pharyngeal wall and lung of a dog
which died with a naturally acquired interstitial pneumonitis (LOU and WENNER,
1963), and from nasal or rectal swabs of four dogs with naturally acquired non-fatal
respiratory disease (MASSIE and SHAW, 1966). In two laboratories (LOU and
WENNER, 1963; MASSIE and SHAW, 1966), experimental infection of puppies
with type 1 strains of canine origin resulted in the appearance of respiratory
illness in all inoculated animals, whereas in another (HOLZINGER and GRIESEMER,
1966), all animals remained well. Interstitial pneumonitis and bronchopneumonia
were observed in one group of experimental animals (LOU and WENNER, 1963)
and cytoplasmic inclusions were seen in the epithelial cells of the bronchial
mucosa of both these animals and the one which died with naturally acquired
disease. In experimental animals, virus was recovered on one or more occasions

from nasal and throat swabs, pharyngeal wall, lung, liver, spleen, and blood (Lou and WENNER, 1963; MASSIE and SHAW, 1966; HOLZINGER and GRIESEMER, 1966). All experimentally infected animals tested at appropriate times were found to have developed homotypic antibody.

e) Other Animals

Naturally occurring disease caused by reoviruses has not been reported from animals other than those mentioned above, but experimentally induced disease has been described in two other species, namely suckling rats (STANLEY et al., 1953) and suckling hamsters (THOMAS et al., 1965). Although no clinical or pathologic manifestations were noted, virus was recovered from the feces of experimentally infected guinea pigs (ROSEN, unpublished) and from the blood of an experimentally infected rabbit (Lou and WENNER, 1963).

No clinical signs were seen in chickens inoculated orally or intravenously with the "Uchida", TS_{17}, or CS_{108} chicken serotypes (KAWAMURA, personal communication). All chicken serotypes produce pocks on the chorio-allantoic membrane of embryonated chicken eggs (KAWAMURA et al., 1965). Seven-day-old eggs are killed by these viruses whether inoculated on the chorio-allantoic membrane or by the yolk-sac or allantoic-cavity routes. Reovirus type 3 has also been shown to multiply on the chorio-allantoic membrane of embryonated chicken eggs, but without causing death of the embryo (STANLEY et al., 1954). Most chicken reoviruses have been recovered from rectal contents or rectal swabs, but on two occasions such viruses were obtained from the trachea (KAWAMURA et al., 1965).

3. Clinical Manifestations, Pathology, and Pathogenesis in Man

The importance of reoviruses as etiologic agents of human disease is still largely unknown. It is obvious that most infections are inapparent or only mildly symptomatic. As judged by serologic surveys (BRICOUT et al., 1965; RUIZ-GOMEZ et al., 1965; SCHMIDT et al., 1965; TAYLOR-ROBINSON, 1965; BROWN and TAYLOR-ROBINSON, 1966; LEERS and ROZEE, 1966; TOTH and HONTY, 1966), human infection with reovirus types 1, 2, and 3 is so common on a world-wide basis that considerable caution must be exercised in attributing an etiologic role to reovirus infections found coinciding in time with various clinical manifestations. The only observed outbreaks of reovirus infection in humans have occurred in institutions for children (ROSEN et al., 1960a, b; MORRONE et al., 1964; STRUTSOVSKAYA et al., 1965) where the prevalence of other microbial agents (BELL et al., 1961) makes it difficult to assess the role of reoviruses as causative factors in the symptomatology observed.

Reovirus isolations have been described from three patients with fatal disease. In one instance, reoviruses were reportedly recovered from two antemortem spinal fluid specimens and from a pool of brain and spinal cord at autopsy from an adult female who died with a disseminated encephalomyelitis (KRAINER and ARONSON, 1959). However, it was not demonstrated conclusively that the viruses were derived from the patient rather than from the test animals, or, that they were reoviruses. The second fatality was a ten-month-old female child who died with an interstitial pneumonitis, myocarditis, hepatitis, and encephalitis (JOSKE et al., 1964). Two strains of reovirus type 1 were isolated in cell culture, one from feces obtained before death and the other from the brain at autopsy. The third fatality was a five-year-old female child who died with a bronchopneumonia (TILLOTSON and LERNER, 1966). Reovirus type 3 was isolated in cell culture from blood, lung, brain, heart, liver, spleen, kidney, adrenal, and lymph node tissue at autopsy. The similarity of the pathologic findings in the latter two cases to those observed in some experimental animals suggest that reoviruses may occasionally cause fatal disease in man.

Concurrent reovirus infection with types 1, 2, or 3 has been demonstrated in children with a great variety of non-fatal illnesses. Clinical manifestations observed include fever, upper and lower tract respiratory disease, gastrointestinal disease, steatorrhea, exanthems, central nervous system disease, and hepatitis (STANLEY et al., 1953; SABIN, 1956; VAN TONGEREN, 1957; RAMOS-ALVAREZ and SABIN, 1958; ROSEN et al., 1960a, b; STANLEY, 1961b; LERNER et al., 1962b; ZALAN et al., 1962a; EL RAI and EVANS, 1963; KELEN et al., 1963; JOSKE et al., 1964; STRUTSOVSKAYA et al., 1965; TURPIN et al., 1965; FANDRE et al., 1966). It does not appear possible at present to determine with any degree of certainty if any of the above illnesses were caused by reoviruses and, consequently, if there are differences in clinical manifestations among the various serotypes. However, in view of the data from the infection of experimental animals, it seems reasonable to suspect that at least some of the clinical manifestations mentioned above, and especially diarrhea and steatorrhea, can indeed be induced by reoviruses.

Reovirus type 1 was isolated from a nasal secretion obtained from an adult with a "common cold" (JACKSON et al., 1962). When this secretion was used to inoculate adult human volunteers, suggestive, but not conclusive, evidence was obtained that the reovirus type 1 in the secretion produced "common colds" in the volunteers. Essentially no illness was produced when the same strain of virus was given to 32 additional volunteers after a number of cell culture passages. Most of the volunteers developed serologic evidence of infection. Similarly, when cell-culture-grown strains of reovirus types 1, 2, or 3 were given to 27 adult volunteers, no illnesses which could be definitely attributed to the inocula were observed (ROSEN et al., 1963b) even though most of the subjects showed virologic and serologic evidence of infection. Neither virologic nor serologic evidence of reovirus infection has been found in a significant proportion of subjects surveyed in studies of upper and lower respiratory tract disease in adults (CHANOCK et al., 1965).

Reoviruses are most commonly recovered from the feces of man, although recovery from the nose or throat is not rare. In longitudinal studies of both naturally and experimentally infected humans (ROSEN et al., 1960a, b, 1963b), reoviruses were recovered much less readily from throat than from rectal swabs. No isolates have been obtained from urine. A four-fold or greater rise in homologous hemagglutination-inhibition antibody has been detected in practically all natural or experimental infections from which appropriate specimens have been available. Individuals with type 3 infections almost always show only a homotypic response, whereas those with type 1 or 2 infections often develop heterotypic antibody (ROSEN et al., 1960a, b, 1963b; KASEL et al., 1963). Hemagglutination-inhibition antibodies are present 21 days after experimental infection in man and may appear earlier. They can be detected for at least one year after natural infection and probably persist much longer.

Reovirus type 3 has been recovered (BELL et al., 1964, 1966) from tumor biopsies from 7 of 31 African patients with Burkitt's lymphoma (BURKITT, 1962). The conditions of virus isolation were such that there seems little doubt that the reoviruses actually were derived from the tumors themselves. However, because of the prevalence and ubiquity of reovirus infections in man, and the known occurrence of reovirus type 3 as a "passenger" agent in mouse tumors, it is difficult to assess the significance of this finding. Obviously, it would be desirable to attempt to isolate viruses by the same methods from the lymphatic tissue of persons who did not have lymphomas but who were matched with lymphoma patients with respect to age, residence, and other factors. Reovirus type 3 was isolated from a normal lymph node as well as from the tumor of one of the lymphoma patients referred to above.

Because of certain epidemiologic characteristics, it has been suggested that Burkitt's lymphoma may be caused by a virus transmitted by arthropods (see BURKITT, 1962). In view of the virus isolations mentioned above, the reports of the isolation of reovirus type 3 from mosquitoes (MILES et al., 1965; L. PARKER et al., 1965), and the alleged similarity of the lymphoma derived from mice inoculated with reovirus type 3 to Burkitt's lymphoma (JOSKE et al., 1966), it has been further hypothesized (STANLEY, 1966a) that Burkitt's lymphoma in Africa is the result of reovirus type 3 infection transmitted to man by mosquitoes from a vertebrate host. This hypothesis is, as yet, unconvincing since each of the observations on which it is based is of uncertain significance.

4. Detection of Infection by Virus Isolation and Serology

Technical aspects of methods for reovirus isolation, identification and serology have been described in detail elsewhere (ROSEN, 1964). This discussion will be limited to general principles and possible sources of error. A few strains of reoviruses have been isolated directly in suckling mice (STANLEY et al., 1953; VAN TONGEREN, 1957; LERNER et al., 1962b), but most have been recovered by the use of cell culture techniques, and the latter are generally considered more sensitive. *Macaca* kidney cell cultures have been the system most widely employed for isolation of reovirus types 1, 2, and 3 and can be considered the system of choice at present. Because of the prevalence of reovirus antibodies in mammalian sera, it is important that the maintenance medium of cell cultures be free of such components. It should also be borne in mind that evidence of endemic infection with reovirus type 3 has been found in most colonies of laboratory mice, and that reovirus type 1 can often be recovered from uninoculated *Macaca* kidney cell cultures maintained for long periods of time. Thus far, reoviruses have not been isolated from uninoculated human embryonic kidney cell cultures, and this is the system of choice when particularly important specimens are to be tested. The use of chicken kidney cell cultures is the only presently known method of isolating chicken reoviruses.

Since the cytopathic effect of reoviruses is slow in appearing when small amounts of virus are inoculated, a "blind" passage is important if one wishes to avoid missing some positive specimens. Although it has been claimed (LERNER et al., 1962a) that this procedure is not necessary when cultures are rolled, experimental data were not presented to substantiate this conclusion. It may be possible to concentrate reovirus type 3 from specimens containing small amounts of virus in a large volume by adsorption to bovine erythrocytes at 4° C (GIBBS and CLIVER, 1965).

Reovirus types 1, 2, and 3 usually can be distinguished from other groups of viruses by the nature of their cytopathic effect in unstained cultures. They are definitively identified and typed by hemagglutination-inhibition techniques using specially prepared or selected type-specific antisera (ROSEN, 1960; BEH-BEHANI et al., 1966). Although difficulty is occasionally encountered in demonstrating agglutination of human erythrocytes by some reovirus preparations, especially with strains of type 3, reports of the absence of this property in particular strains have not been confirmed.

Most serologic investigations involving reovirus types 1, 2, and 3 have employed hemagglutination-inhibition tests. Not only is this procedure simpler in general than either the neutralization or the complement-fixation test, but the latter two procedures are also less satisfactory in this case for the following reasons. In the neutralization test, a relatively large amount of test virus is required in order to obtain a cytopathic effect before the cell cultures degenerate spontaneously. Consequently, small amounts of antibody are difficult to detect. In the complement-fixation test, it is not possible to detect complement-fixing antibodies in many post-infection sera. In other words, both tests are less sensitive than the hemagglutination-inhibition test. When complement-fixing antibodies are present, they are apparently group- rather than type-specific (SABIN, 1959). Since reovirus antibodies are very common in sera of all types, it is essential that paired sera be employed for diagnostic purposes. Because of the antigenic heterogeneity of type 2 strains, it may be necessary to employ more than one antigen for serologic tests with this type. If available, an antigen prepared from a homologous isolate would be the most satisfactory. This procedure has not been found to be necessary for types 1 or 3.

A micro-neutralization test has been developed (SCHMIDT et al., 1966) for reoviruses which is said to be more *specific* than the hemagglutination-inhibition test with animal sera. This conclusion was based on the observation that no neutralizing antibody was found in some sera which had hemagglutination-inhibition antibody. However, it is also possible to interpret the data as indicating that the neutralization is less *sensitive* than the hemagglutination-inhibition test.

VII. Interaction with Groups of Organisms (Epidemiology)

Perhaps the most striking aspect of the epidemiology of reoviruses is that, with the exception of the chicken serotypes, strains which have been recovered from a wide variety of lower animals are indistinguishable from each other and from those which have been isolated from man (ROSEN, 1962). While it is not unusual for a few species to share identical viruses, or for many species to share *related* viruses (e.g. adenoviruses), the situation with respect to reoviruses is unique. The occurrence of identical viruses in different species naturally suggests the possibility of transmission from one species to another in nature. Although, such transmission has not been demonstrated, it is almost inconceivable that it does not occur on occasion. In view of the similarities of certain leafhopper-borne viruses affecting plants to reoviruses and the great variety of such agents known, it is tempting to speculate that plant or non-bloodsucking insect hosts of reoviruses may also exist.

There is considerable evidence that the epidemiology of reovirus types 1, 2, and 3 is not identical. For example, although reovirus type 3 is apparently very prevalent in mouse colonies (ROWE et al., 1962) types 1 and 2 have never been recovered from such animals — although the latter type has been isolated from wild mice. Similarly, in all instances where typing has been attempted, reoviruses isolated from uninoculated *Macaca* or *Cercopithecus* kidney cell cultures have been identified as type 1. On the other hand, all three types have been recovered from cattle. There are no data to suggest that any particular serotype is more or less prevalent than another in any particular geographic area.

It appears that reovirus infections are usually acquired relatively early in life. Thus, most strains isolated from humans have come from children and in a longitudinal study of three dairy herds (ROSEN et al., 1963a) almost every calf was infected with at least one serotype by the age of one year.

Reoviruses are found most frequently in the feces of naturally infected lower animals and man, and it is logical to suspect that the primary means of transmission is by the fecal-oral route. Of course, in view of the known respiratory manifestations of reovirus infections, transmission to or from the respiratory tract may occur, but evidence to this effect is lacking. Despite the possible recovery of reoviruses from mosquitoes, there is no evidence as yet to suggest transmission by an arthropod vector. There is also no evidence for transplacental transmission under natural conditions.

Outbreaks of infection with reovirus types 1, 2, and 3 in institutions for children have occurred in late summer, fall, and winter (ROSEN et al., 1960a, b; STRUTSOVSKAYA et al., 1965). In one community study (GELFAND, 1959), most reovirus isolates were obtained in the winter, whereas in another (GELFAND et al., 1963), most were obtained in the summer and fall. In a longitudinal study of dairy cattle (ROSEN et al., 1963a) most reovirus infections occurred in the fall and winter. It is also of interest to note that the recovery of reovirus type 1 from uninoculated *Macaca* kidney cell cultures occurred commonly only in winter (January, February, and March) of two successive years (HULL and MINNER, 1957).

References

ACS, G., E. REICH, and M. MORI: Biological and biochemical properties of the analogue antibiotic tubercidin. Proc. nat. Acad. Sci. (Wash.) 52, 493—501 (1964).

ALLISON, A. C., F. E. BUCKLAND, and C. H. ANDREWES: Effects of sulfhydryl reagents on infectivity of some viruses. Virology 17, 171—175 (1962).

ARNOTT, S., F. HUTCHINSON, M. SPENCER, M. H. F. WILKINS, W. FULLER, and R. LANGRIDGE: X-ray diffraction studies of double helical ribonucleic acid. Nature (Lond.) 211, 227—232 (1966).

BEHBEHANI, A. M., L. C. FOSTER, and H. A. WENNER: Preparation of type-specific antisera to reoviruses. Appl. Microbiol. 14, 1051—1053 (1966).

BELL, T. M.: An Introduction to General Virology, p. 99. J. B. Lippincott Co., Phila.,
1965.
BELL, J. A., R. J. HUEBNER, L. ROSEN, W. P. ROWE, R. M. COLE, F. M. MASTROTA,
T. M. FLOYD, R. M. CHANOCK, and R. A. SHVEDOFF: Illness and microbial experiences of nursery children at junior village. Amer. J. Hyg. 74, 267—292 (1961).
BELL, T. M., A. MASSIE, M. G. R. ROSS, D. I. H. SIMPSON, and E. GRIFFIN: Further
isolations of reovirus type 3 from cases of Burkitt's lymphoma. Brit. med. J. I,
1514—1517 (1966).
BELL, T. M., A. MASSIE, M. G. R. ROSS, and M. C. WILLIAMS: Isolation of a reovirus
from a case of Burkitt's lymphoma. Brit. med. J. I, 1212—1213 (1964).
BENNETTE, J. G.: Isolation of a non-pathogenic tumor-destroying virus from mouse
ascites. Nature (Lond.) 187, 72—73 (1960).
BENO, D. W., and E. A. EDWARDS: Formalinized red cells in diagnostic virology.
Publ. Hth. Rep. (Wash.) 81, 377—381 (1966).
BERNHARD, W., and N. GRANBOULAN: Morphology of oncogenic and non-oncogenic
mouse viruses, in "CIBA Foundation Symposium on Tumour Viruses of Murine
Origin" (WOLSTENHOLME and O'CONNOR, eds.) pp. 6—49. Little, Brown and
Co., Boston, 1962.
BERNHARD, W., and P. TOURNIER: Ultrastructural cytochemistry applied to the
study of virus infection, Cold Spr. Harb. Symp. quant. Biol., 27, 67—82 (1962).
BILS, R. F., and C. E. HALL: Electron microscopy of wound-tumor virus. Virology 17,
123—130 (1962).
BLACK, L. M.: Some viruses transmitted by agallian leafhoppers. Proc. Amer. Philosoph.
Soc. 88, 132—144 (1944).
BLACK, L. M.: Occasional transmission of some plant viruses through the eggs of
their insect vectors. Phytopathology 43, 9—10 (1953).
BLACK, L. M.: Biological cycles of plant viruses in insect vectors, in "The Viruses"
(BURNET and STANLEY, eds.), vol. 2, pp. 157—185. Academic Press, New York—
London, 1959.
BLACK, L. M.: Physiology of virus-induced tumors in plants, in "Handbuch der
Pflanzen-Physiologie" (RUHLAND, ed.), vol. 15, pp. 236—266. Springer, Heidel-
berg, 1965.
BLACK, L. M., and R. MARKHAM: Base-pairing in the ribonucleic acid of wound-tumor
virus. Neth. J. Plant Path. 69, 215 (1963).
BRICOUT, F., J. REGNARD et J. DUVAL: Pouvoir pathogène et diffusion des réo-
virus. Ann. Pédiat. 41, 43—48 (1965).
BROWN, P. K., and D. TAYLOR-ROBINSON: Respiratory virus antibodies in sera of
persons living in isolated communities. Bull. Wld Hlth Org. 34, 895—900 (1966).
BRUBAKER, M. M., B. WEST, and R. J. ELLIS: Human blood group influence on
reovirus hemagglutination titers. Proc. Soc. exp. Biol. (N.Y.) 115, 1118—1120
(1964).
BUCKLAND, F. E.: Impairment of viral haemagglutination of red cells after treatment
with formalin. Nature (Lond.) 183, 1276 (1959).
BUCKLAND, F. E.: Inactivation of virus haemagglutinins by para-chloromercuribenzoic
acid. Nature (Lond.) 188, 768 (1960).
BUCKLAND, F. E., and D. A. J. TYRRELL: A comparative study of virus haemagglutinins. The stability of haemagglutinins and red cell receptors to certain physical
and chemical treatments. J. gen. Microbiol. 32, 241—253 (1963).
BURKITT, D.: A tumor syndrome affecting children in tropical Africa. Postgrad.
med. J. 38, 71—79 (1962).
CASALS, J., and D. H. CLARKE: Arboviruses other than groups A and B, in "Viral
and Rickettsial Infections of Man" (HORSFALL and TAMM, eds.), 4th ed., pp. 659—
684. J. B. Lippincott Co., Phila.—Montreal, 1965.
CHANOCK, R. M., M. A. MUFSON, and K. M. JOHNSON: Comparative biology and
ecology of human virus and mycoplasma respiratory pathogens. Progr. med.
Virol. 7, 208—252 (1965).

Committee on the ECHO Viruses: Enteric cytopathogenic human orphan (ECHO) viruses. Science **122**, 1187—1188 (1955).

COOK, I.: Reovirus type 3 infection in laboratory mice. Aust. J. exp. Biol. med. Sci. **41**, 651—659 (1963).

DALES, S.: Association between the spindle apparatus and reovirus. Proc. nat. Acad. Sci. (Wash.) **50**, 268—275 (1963).

DALES, S.: Effects of streptovitacin A on the initial events in the replication of vaccinia and reovirus. Proc. nat. Acad. Sci. (Wash.) **54**, 462—468 (1965).

DALES, S., P. J. GOMATOS, and K. C. HSU: The uptake and development of reovirus in strain L cells followed with labeled viral ribonucleic acid and ferritin-antibody conjugates. Virology **25**, 193—211 (1965).

DARDANONI, L., e P. ZAFFIRO: Sul potere emoagglutinante di virus appartenenti al gruppo ECHO. Boll. Ist. sieroter. milan. **37**, 346—350 (1958).

DROUHET, V.: Sur l'effet cytopathogène du virus ECHO 10. Ann. Inst. Pasteur **95**, 781—784 (1958).

DROUHET, V.: Lésions cellulaires provoquées par les réovirus (virus ECHO 10). Anticorps fluorescents et étude cytochimique. Ann. Inst. Pasteur **98**, 618—621 (1960).

EGGERS, H. J., P. J. GOMATOS, and I. TAMM: Agglutination of bovine erythrocytes: A general characteristic of reovirus type 3. Proc. Soc. exp. Biol. (N.Y.) **110**, 879—881 (1962).

EGGERS, H. J., and I. TAMM: Spectrum and characteristics of the virus inhibitory action of 2-(α-hydroxybenzyl)-benzimidazole. J. exp. Med. **113**, 657—682 (1961).

EL-RAI, F. M., and A. S. EVANS: Reovirus infections in children and young adults. Arch. environm. Hlth. **7**, 700—704 (1963).

FANDRE, M., G. DROPSY, R. COFFIN, F. PENNAFORTE et J. BOCHET: Les bronchiolites aigües virales du nourrisson. Pédiatrie **21**, 545—557 (1966).

FOUAD, M. T. A., and R. ENGLER: Density gradient centrifugation of reovirus prototypes 1, 2 and 3. Z. Naturforsch. **21b**, 706—707 (1966).

FRANKLIN, R. M.: Comparison of assays for mengovirus and reovirus 3. Proc. Soc. exp. Biol. (N.Y.) **107**, 651—653 (1961).

FUKUSHI, T., and E. SHIKATA: Fine structure of rice dwarf virus. Virology **21**, 500—503 (1963a).

FUKUSHI, T., and E. SHIKATA: Localization of rice dwarf virus in its insect vector. Virology **21**, 503—505 (1963b).

FUKUSHI, T., E. SHIKATA, and I. KIMURA: Some morphological characters of rice dwarf virus. Virology **18**, 192—205 (1962).

GELB, L. D., and A. M. LERNER: Reovirus hemagglutination: Inhibition by N-acetyl-D-glucosamine. Science **147**, 404—405 (1965).

GELFAND, H. M.: The incidence of certain endemic enteric virus infections in Southern Louisiana. Sth. med. J. **52**, 819—827 (1959).

GELFAND, H. M., A. H. HOLGUIN, G. E. MARCHETTI, and P. M. FEORINO: A continuing surveillance of enterovirus infections in healthy children in six United States cities. I. Viruses isolated during 1960 and 1961. Amer. J. Hyg. **78**, 358—375 (1963).

GIBBS, T., and D. O. CLIVER: Methods for detecting minimal contamination with reovirus. Hlth Lab. Sci. **2**, 81—88 (1965).

GOLDFIELD, M., S. SRIHONGSE, and J. P. FOX: Hemagglutinins associated with certain human enteric viruses. Proc. Soc. exp. Biol. (N.Y.) **96**, 788—791 (1957).

GOMATOS, P. J., R. M. KRUG, and I. TAMM: Enzymic synthesis of RNA with reovirus RNA as template. I. Characteristics of the reaction catalyzed by the RNA polymerase from *Escherichia coli*. J. molec. Biol. **9**, 193—207 (1964).

GOMATOS, P. J., R. M. KRUG, and I. TAMM: Reovirus RNA-directed synthesis of DNA. I. The reaction catalyzed by DNA polymerase from *Escherichia coli*. J. molec. Biol. **13**, 802—816 (1965).

GOMATOS, P. J., and W. STOECKENIUS: Electron microscope studies on reovirus RNA. Proc. nat. Acad. Sci. (Wash.) **52**, 1449—1455 (1964).

GOMATOS, P. J., and I. TAMM: Reactive sites of reovirus type 3 and their interaction with receptor substances. Virology 17, 455—461 (1962).

GOMATOS, P. J., and I. TAMM: The secondary structure of reovirus RNA. Proc. nat. Acad. Sci. (Wash.) 49, 707—714 (1963a).

GOMATOS, P. J., and I. TAMM: Animal and plant viruses with double-helical RNA. Proc. nat. Acad. Sci. (Wash.) 50, 878—885 (1963b).

GOMATOS, P. J., and I. TAMM: Base composition of the RNA of a reovirus variant. Science 140, 997—998 (1963c).

GOMATOS, P. J., and I. TAMM: Macromolecular synthesis in reovirus-infected L cells. Biochim. biophys. Acta (Amst.) 72, 651—653 (1963d).

GOMATOS, P. J., I. TAMM, S. DALES, and R. M. FRANKLIN: Reovirus type 3: Physical characteristics and interaction with L cells. Virology 17, 441—454 (1962).

GROSE, F. J., M. H. BERNSTEIN, and A. M. LERNER: 'Ring-forms' of reovirus particles. Nature (Lond.) 208, 606—607 (1965).

HALONEN, P.: Growth, stability and hemagglutination of a reovirus. Ann. Med. exp. Fenn. 39, 132—142 (1961).

HALONEN, P., and M. PYHTILA: Purification of reovirus and measles virus hemagglutinin by fluorocarbon, on calcium phosphate and by differential gradient centrifugation. Ann. Med. exp. Fenn. 40, 365—376 (1962).

HARFORD, C. G., A. HAMLIN, J. N. MIDDELKAMP, and D. D. BRIGGS, JR.: Electron microscopic examination of cells infected with reovirus. J. Lab. clin. Med. 60, 179—193 (1962).

HARTLEY, J. W., W. P. ROWE, and J. B. AUSTIN: Subtype differentiation of reovirus type 2 strains by hemagglutination-inhibition with mouse antisera. Virology 16, 94—96 (1962).

HARTLEY, J. W., W. P. ROWE, and R. J. HUEBNER: Recovery of reoviruses from wild and laboratory mice. Proc. Soc. exp. Biol. (N.Y.) 108, 390—395 (1961).

HASHIMI, A., M. M. CARRUTHERS, P. WOLF, and A. M. LERNER: Congenital infections with reovirus. J. exp. Med. 124, 33—46 (1966).

HASSAN, S. A., and K. W. COCHRAN: Teratogenicity of reo- and poliovirus in mice. Bact. Proc., p. 115 (1966).

HASSAN, S. A., E. R. RABIN, and J. L. MELNICK: Reovirus myocarditis in mice: An electron microscopic, immunofluorescent, and virus assay study. Exp. molec. Path. 4, 66—80 (1965).

HAYASHI, Y., and S. KAWASE: Base pairing in ribonucleic acid extracted from the cytoplasmic polyhedra of the silkworm. Virology 23, 611—614 (1964).

HAYASHI, Y., and S. KAWASE: Studies on the RNA in the cytoplasmic polyhedra of the silkworm, Bombyx mori L. (II) Base composition of the specific RNA extracted from cytoplasmic polyhedra. J. sericult. Sci. Japan 34, 90—94 (1965). (In Japanese).

HIATT, C. W.: Photodynamic inactivation of viruses. Trans. N.Y. Acad. Sci. 23, 66—78 (1960).

HOBBS, T. R., and C. C. MASCOLI: Studies on experimental infection of weanling mice with reoviruses. Proc. Soc. exp. Biol. (N.Y.) 118, 847—853 (1965).

HOLZINGER, E. A., and R. A. GRIESEMER: Effects of reovirus, type 1, on germfree and disease-free dogs. Amer. J. Epidem. 84, 426—430 (1966).

HOWELL, P. G.: The isolation and identification of further antigenic types of African horsesickness virus. Onderstepoort J. vet. Res. 29, 139—149 (1962).

HSIUNG, G. D.: Some distinctive biological characteristics of ECHO-10 virus. Proc. Soc. exp. Biol. (N.Y.) 99, 387—390 (1958).

HULL, R. N., and J. R. MINNER: New viral agents recovered from tissue cultures of monkey kidney cells. II. Problems of isolation and identification. Ann. N.Y. Acad. Sci. 67, 413—423 (1957).

HULL, R. N., J. R. MINNER, and C. C. MASCOLI: New viral agents recovered from tissue cultures of monkey kidney cells. III. Recovery of additional agents both from cultures of monkey tissues and directly from tissues and excreta. Amer. J. Hyg. 68, 31—44 (1958).

HULL, R. N., J. R. MINNER, and J. W. SMITH: New viral agents recovered from tissue cultures of monkey kidney cells. I. Origin and properties of cytopathogenic agents $S.V._1$, $S.V._2$, $S.V._4$, $S.V._5$, $S.V._6$, $S.V._{11}$, $S.V._{12}$, and $S.V._{15}$. Amer. J. Hyg. 63, 204—215 (1956).

JACKSON, G. G., R. L. MULDOON, G. C. JOHNSON, and H. F. DOWLING: Contributions of volunteers to studies on the common cold. Amer. Rev. resp. Dis. 88 (part 2), 120—127 (1962).

JENSON, A. B., E. R. RABIN, C. A. PHILLIPS, and J. L. MELNICK: Reovirus encephalitis in newborn mice. Amer. J. Path. 47, 223—239 (1965).

JONCAS, J.: The direct fluorescent antibody technique studied with reovirus type 1. Rev. Canad. Biol. 23, 333—338 (1964).

JORDAN, L. E., and H. D. MAYOR: The fine structure of reovirus, a new member of the icosahedral series. Virology 17, 597—599 (1962).

JOSKE, R. A., D. D. KEALL, P. J. LEAK, N. F. STANLEY, and M. N.-I. WALTERS: Hepatitis-encephalitis in humans with reovirus infection. Arch. intern. Med. 113, 811—816 (1964).

JOSKE, R. A., P. J. LEAK, J. M. PAPADIMITRIOU, N. F. STANLEY, and M. N.-I. WALTERS: Murine infection with reovirus: IV. Late chronic disease and the induction of lymphoma after reovirus type 3 infection. Brit. J. exp. Path. 47, 337—346 (1966).

KASEL, J. A., L. ROSEN, and H. E. EVANS: Infection of human volunteers with a reovirus of bovine origin. Proc. Soc. exp. Biol. (N.Y.) 112, 979—981 (1963).

KAWAMURA, H., F. SHIMIZU, M. MAEDA, and H. TSUBAHARA: Avian reovirus: Its properties and serological classification. Nat. Inst. Anim. Hlth. quart. 5, 115—124 (1965).

KAWAMURA, H., and H. TSUBAHARA: Common antigenicity of avian reoviruses. Nat. Inst. Anim. Hlth. quart. 6, 187—193 (1966).

KEAST, D., and N. F. STANLEY: Studies on a murine lymphoma induced by reovirus type 3: Some general aspects of the lymphoma 2731/L. Proc. Soc. exp. Biol. (N.Y.) 122, 1091—1098 (1966).

KELEN, A. E., D. BELBIN, J. M. LESIAK, and N. A. LABZOFFSKY: Isolation of enteric viruses in Ontario during 1960—1962. Canad. med. Ass. J. 89, 921—926 (1963).

KETLER, A., V. V. HAMPARIAN, and M. R. HILLEMAN: Characterization and classification of ECHO 28-rhinovirus-coryzavirus agents. Proc. Soc. exp. Biol. (N.Y.) 110, 821—831 (1962).

KLEIN, P. A.: Antibody-mediated immunity to transplantable tumors following reovirus oncolysis. Path. Microbiol. In press (1967).

KLEINSCHMIDT, A. K., T. H. DUNNEBACKE, R. S. SPENDLOVE, F. L. SCHAFFER, and R. F. WHITCOMB: Electron microscopy of RNA from reovirus and wound tumor virus. J. molec. Biol. 10, 282—288 (1964).

KRAINER, L., and B. E. ARONSON: Disseminated encephalomyelitis in the human with recovery of hepatoencephalitis virus (HEV); pathologic and virologic report. J. Neuropath. exp. Neurol. 18, 339—342 (1959).

KRUG, R. M., P. J. GOMATOS, and I. TAMM: Enzymic synthesis of RNA with reovirus RNA as template. II. Nearest neighbor analysis of the products of the reaction catalyzed by the *Escherichia coli* RNA polymerase. J. molec. Biol. 12, 872—880 (1965).

KUDO, H., and A. F. GRAHAM: Synthesis of reovirus ribonucleic acid in L cells. J. Bact. 90, 936—945 (1965).

KUDO, H., and A. F. GRAHAM: Selective inhibition of reovirus induced RNA in L cells. Biochem. biophys. Res. Commun. 24, 150—155 (1966).

KUNDIN, W. D., C. LIU, and J. GIGSTAD: Reovirus infection in suckling mice: Immunofluorescent and infectivity studies. J. Immunol. 97, 393—401 (1966).

LAMONT, P. H.: Some bovine respiratory viruses. Proc. roy. Soc. Med. 59, 50—51 (1966).

LANGRIDGE, R., and P. J. GOMATOS: The structure of RNA. Reovirus RNA and transfer RNA have similar three-dimensional structures, which differ from DNA. Science 141, 694—698 (1963).

LA PLACA, M.: Electron microscope study of a reovirus-related strain, of bovine origin, in ultrathin sections of monkey kidney infected cells. G. Microbiol. **10**, 111—115 (1962).

LEERS, W. D., and K. R. ROZEE: A survey of reovirus antibodies in sera of urban children. Canad. med. Ass. J. **94**, 1040—1042 (1966).

LENAHAN, M. F., and H. A. WENNER: Propagation of entero- and other viruses in renal cells obtained from non-primate hosts. J. infect. Dis. **107**, 203—212 (1960).

LERNER, A. M., E. J. BAILEY, and M. KOFENDER: Preparations of saliva inhibiting reovirus hemagglutination. J. Immunol. **96**, 59—63 (1966).

LERNER, A. M., E. J. BAILEY, and J. R. TILLOTSON: Enterovirus hemagglutination: Inhibition by several enzymes and sugars. J. Immunol. **95**, 1111—1115 (1965).

LERNER, A. M., J. D. CHERRY, and M. FINLAND: Enhancement of cytopathic effects of reoviruses in rolled cultures of rhesus kidney. Proc. Soc. exp. Biol. (N.Y.) **110**, 727—729 (1962).

LERNER, A. M., J. D. CHERRY, and M. FINLAND: Hemagglutination with reoviruses. Virology **19**, 58—65 (1963).

LERNER, A. M., J. D. CHERRY, J. O. KLEIN, and M. FINLAND: Infections with reoviruses. New Engl. J. Med. **267**, 947—952 (1962).

LERNER, A. M., L. D. GELB, J. R. TILLOTSON, M. M. CARRUTHERS, and E. J. BAILEY: Enterovirus hemagglutination: Inhibition by aldoses and a possible mechanism. J. Immunol. **96**, 629—636 (1966).

LIVINGSTON, C. W., JR., and R. W. MOORE: Cytochemical changes of bluetongue virus in tissue cultures. Amer. J. vet. Res. **23**, 701—710 (1962).

LOH, P. C., H. R. HOHL, and M. SOERGEL: Fine structure of reovirus type 2. J. Bact. **89**, 1140—1144 (1965).

LOH, P. C., and M. SOERGEL: Growth characteristics of reovirus type 2: Actinomycin D and the synthesis of viral RNA. Proc. nat. Acad. Sci. (Wash.) **54**, 857—863 (1965).

LOH, P. C., and M. SOERGEL: Growth characteristics of reovirus type 2: Actinomycin D and the preferential synthesis of viral RNA. Proc. Soc. exp. Biol. (N.Y.) **122**, 1248—1250 (1966).

LOH, P. C., and M. SOERGEL: Macromolecular synthesis in cells infected with reovirus type 2 and the effect of Ara-C. Nature. **214**, 622—623 (1967).

LOU, T. Y., and H. A. WENNER: Natural and experimental infection of dogs with reovirus, type 1: Pathogenicity of the strain for other animals. Amer. J. Hyg. **77**, 293—304 (1963).

MALHERBE, H., and R. HARWIN: Seven viruses isolated from the vervet monkey. Brit. J. exp. Path. **38**, 539—541 (1957).

MALHERBE, H., R. HARWIN, and M. ULRICH: The cytopathic effects of vervet monkey viruses. S. Afr. med. J. **37**, 407—411 (1963).

MARAMOROSCH, K.: Arthropod transmission of plant viruses. Ann. Rev. Entom. **8**, 369—414 (1963).

MARAMOROSCH, K.: Interrelationships between plant pathogenic viruses and insects. Ann. N.Y.Acad. Sci. **118**, 363—370 (1964).

MASSIE, E. L., and E. D. SHAW: Reovirus type 1 in laboratory dogs. Amer. J. vet. Res. **27**, 783—787 (1966).

MAYOR, H. D.: Studies on reovirus. III. A labile, single-stranded ribonucleic acid associated with the late stages of infection. J. nat. Cancer Inst. **35**, 919—925 (1965).

MAYOR, H. D., R. M. JAMISON, L. E. JORDAN, and M. VAN MITCHELL: Reoviruses. II. Structure and composition of the virion. J. Bact. **89**, 1548—1556 (1965).

MAYOR, H. D., and L. E. JORDAN: Studies on reovirus. I. Morphologic observations on the development of reovirus in tissue culture. Exp. molec. Path. **4**, 40—50 (1965).

MCCLAIN, M. E., and R. S. SPENDLOVE: Multiplicity reactivation of reovirus particles after exposure to ultraviolet light. J. Bact. **92**, 1422—1429 (1966).

MCCLAIN, M. E., R. S. SPENDLOVE, and E. H. LENNETTE: Infectivity assay of reoviruses: Comparison of immunofluorescent cell count and plaque methods. J. Immunol. **98**, 1301—1308 (1967).

MELNICK, J. L., W. C. COCKBURN, G. DALLDORF, S. GARD, J. H. S. GEAR, W. McD. HAMMON, M. M. KAPLAN, F. P. NAGLER, N. OKER-BLOM, A. J. RHODES, A. B. SABIN, J. D. VERLINDE, and H. VON MAGNUS: Picornavirus group. Virology 19, 114—116 (1963).

MILES, J. A. R., F. J. AUSTIN, F. N. MACNAMARA, and T. MAGUIRE: Isolation of reovirus type 3 from mosquitoes and from bird bloods from South Westland. Proc. Univ. Otago med. Sch. 43, 27—29 (1965).

MIURA, K.-I., I. KIMURA, and N. SUZUKI: Double-stranded ribonucleic acid from rice dwarf virus. Virology 28, 571—579 (1966).

MORRONE, G., L. DARDANONI, N. DE CICCO e C. SPANO: Su un episodio epidemico riferibile ad infezione da reovirus. Pediatria (Napoli) 72, 254—265 (1964).

MOSCOVICI, C., M. LA PLACA, J. MAISEL, and C. H. KEMPE: Studies of bovine enteroviruses. Amer. J. vet. Res. 22, 852—863 (1961).

MÜLLER, G., C. C. SCHNEIDER, and D. PETERS: Zur Feinstruktur des Reovirus (Typ 3). Arch. ges. Virusforsch. 19, 110—122 (1966).

NELSON, J. B.: Response of mice to reovirus type 3 in presence and absence of ascites tumor cells. Proc. Soc. exp. Biol. (N.Y.) 116, 1086—1089 (1964).

NELSON, J. B., and G. R. COLLINS: The establishment and maintenance of a specific pathogen-free colony of Swiss mice. Proc. animal Care Panel 11, 65—72 (1961).

NELSON, J. B., and G. S. TARNOWSKI: An oncolytic virus recovered from Swiss mice during passage of an ascites tumour. Nature (Lond.) 188, 886—887 (1960).

NEWLIN, S. C., and A. P. McKEE: Erythrocyte receptor specificity of reovirus isolates. Bact. Proc., p. 127 (1966).

OIE, H., P. C. LOH, and M. SOERGEL: Growth characteristics and immunocytochemical studies of reovirus type 2 in a line of human amnion cells. Arch. ges. Virusforsch. 18, 16—24 (1966).

PAPADIMITRIOU, J. M.: Electron micrographic features of acute murine reovirus hepatitis. Amer. J. Path. 47, 565—585 (1965).

PAPADIMITRIOU, J. M.: Electron microscopic findings of a murine lymphoma associated with reovirus type 3 infection. Proc. Soc. exp. Biol. (N.Y.) 121, 93—96 (1966).

PARKER, J. C., R. W. TENNANT, and T. G. WARD: Prevalence of viruses in mouse colonies, in "Viruses of Laboratory Rodents" (HOLDENRIED, ed.), National Cancer Institute Monograph 20, pp. 25—36, 1966.

PARKER, J. C., R. W. TENNANT, T. G. WARD, and W. P. ROWE: Virus studies with germfree mice. I. Preparation of serologic diagnostic reagents and survey of germfree and monocontaminated mice for indigenous murine viruses. J. nat. Cancer Inst. 34, 371—380 (1965).

PARKER, L., E. BAKER, and N. F. STANLEY: The isolation of reovirus type 3 from mosquitoes and a sentinel infant mouse. Aust. J. exp. Biol. med. Sci. 43, 167—170 (1965).

POLSON, A., and D. DEEKS: Electron microscopy of neurotropic African horsesickness virus. J. Hyg. (Lond.) 61, 149—153 (1963).

PREVEC, L., and A. F. GRAHAM: Reovirus-specific polyribosomes in infected L-cells. Science 154, 522—523 (1966).

RAMOS-ALVAREZ, M., and A. B. SABIN: Characteristics of poliomyelitis and other enteric viruses recovered in tissue culture from healthy American children. Proc. Soc. exp. Biol. (N.Y.) 87, 655—661 (1954).

RAMOS-ALVAREZ, M., and A. B. SABIN: Intestinal viral flora of healthy children demonstrable by monkey kidney tissue culture. Amer. J. publ. Hlth 46, 295—299 (1956).

RAMOS-ALVAREZ, M., and A. B. SABIN: Enteropathogenic viruses and bacteria. Role in summer diarrheal diseases of infancy and early childhood. J. Amer. med. Ass. 167, 147—156 (1958).

RAUTH, A. M.: The physical state of viral nucleic acid and the sensitivity of viruses to ultraviolet light. Biophys. J. 5, 257—273 (1965).

RHIM, J. S., L. E. JORDAN, and H. D. MAYOR: Cytochemical, fluorescent-antibody and electron microscopic studies on the growth of reovirus (ECHO 10) in tissue culture. Virology 17, 342—355 (1962).

RHIM, J. S., J. I. KATO, and W. PELON: Hemagglutination by reoviruses propagated in various cell lines. Proc. Soc. exp. Biol. (N.Y.) 118, 453—459 (1965).

RHIM, J. S., and J. L. MELNICK: Plaque formation by reoviruses. Virology 15, 80—81 (1961a).

RHIM, J. S., and J. L. MELNICK: Quantitative studies of reovirus (ECHO 10) in monkey kidney cell cultures. Tex. Rep. Biol. Med. 19, 851—859 (1961b).

RHIM, J. S., K. O. SMITH, and J. L. MELNICK: Complete and coreless forms of reovirus (ECHO 10). Ratio of number of virus particles to infective units in the one-step growth cycle. Virology 15, 428—435 (1961).

RIGHTSEL, W. A., J. R. DICE, R. J. McALPINE, E. A. TIMM, I. W. McLEAN, JR., G. J. DIXON, and F. M. SCHABEL, JR.: Antiviral effect of guanidine. Science 134, 558—559 (1961).

ROSEN, L.: Serologic grouping of reoviruses by hemagglutination-inhibition. Amer. J. Hyg. 71, 242—249 (1960).

ROSEN, L.: Reoviruses in animals other than man. Ann. N.Y. Acad. Sci. 101, 461—465 (1962).

ROSEN, L.: Reoviruses, in "Diagnostic Procedures for Viral and Rickettsial Diseases' (LENNETTE and SCHMIDT, eds.), pp. 259—267. Amer. Public Health Association, Inc., New York, 1964.

ROSEN, L., and F. R. ABINANTI: Natural and experimental infection of cattle with human types of reoviruses. Amer. J. Hyg. 71, 250—257 (1960).

ROSEN, L., F. R. ABINANTI, and J. F. HOVIS: Further observations on the natural infection of cattle with reoviruses. Amer. J. Hyg. 77, 38—48 (1963).

ROSEN, L., H. E. EVANS, and A. SPICKARD: Reovirus infections in human volunteers. Amer. J. Hyg. 77, 29—37 (1963).

ROSEN, L., J. F. HOVIS, F. M. MASTROTA, J. A. BELL, and R. J. HUEBNER: Observations on a newly recognized virus (Abney) of the reovirus family. Amer. J. Hyg. 71, 258—265 (1960a).

ROSEN, L., J. F. HOVIS, F. M. MASTROTA, J. A. BELL, and R. J. HUEBNER: An outbreak of infection with a type 1 reovirus among children in an institution. Amer. J. Hyg. 71, 266—274 (1960b).

ROSSER, J. M., I. S. JOHNSON, H. F. WRIGHT, and D. H. HOLMES: Biological and physical characteristics of an oncolytic virus isolated from mouse ascites cells. J. Cell Biol. 27, 90A—91A (1965).

ROWE, W. P., J. W. HARTLEY, and R. J. HUEBNER: Polyoma and other indigenous mouse viruses, in "The Problems of Laboratory Animal Disease" (HARRIS, ed.), pp. 131—142. Academic Press, London—New York, 1962.

RUIZ-GOMEZ, J., I. FAINGEZICHT-GUTMAN y J. SOSA-MARTINEZ: Virus reo: Investigación de anticuerpos en individuos de diferentes edades. Bol. méd. Hosp. infant (Méx.) 22, 359—363 (1965).

SABIN, A. B.: The significance of viruses recovered from the intestinal tracts of healthy infants and children. Ann. N.Y. Acad. Sci. 66, 226—230 (1956).

SABIN, A. B.: Reoviruses: A new group of respiratory and enteric viruses formerly classified as ECHO type 10 is described. Science 130, 1387—1389 (1959).

SABIN, A. B.: Role of ECHO viruses in human disease, in "Viral Infections of Infancy and Childhood" (ROSE, ed.), pp. 78—100. Hoeber-Harper, New York, 1960.

SAFFERMAN, R. S., and M.-E. MORRIS: Algal virus: Isolation. Science 140, 679—680 (1963).

SATO, T., Y. KYOGOKU, S. HIGUCHI, Y. MITSUI, Y. IITAKA, M. TSUBOI, and K.-I. MIURA: A preliminary investigation on the molecular structure of rice dwarf virus ribonucleic acid. J. molec. Biol. 16, 180—190 (1966).

SATTAR, S. A., and K. R. ROZEE: Studies on the biological properties and classification of SV_4 virus. Canad. J. Microbiol. 11, 325—335 (1965).

SCHMIDT, J., C. TAUCHNITZ, and O. KUHN: Untersuchungen über das Vorkommen hämagglutinationshemmender Antikörper gegen die Reovirustypen 1 und 2 in der Bevölkerung. Z. Hyg. Infekt.-Kr. 150, 269—279 (1965).

SCHMIDT, N. J., J. DENNIS, M. N. HOFFMAN, and E. H. LENNETTE: Inhibitors of echovirus and reovirus hemagglutination. I. Inhibitors in tissue culture fluids. J. Immunol. 93, 367—376 (1964a).

SCHMIDT, N. J., J. DENNIS, M. N. HOFFMAN, and E. H. LENNETTE: Inhibitors of echovirus and reovirus hemagglutination. II. Serum and phospholipid inhibitors. J. Immunol. 93, 377—386 (1964b).

SCHMIDT, N. J., J. DENNIS, and E. H. LENNETTE: Studies on filtrates from cultures of a psychrophylic *Pseudomonas* sp. which inactivate nonspecific serum inhibitors for certain hemagglutinating viruses. J. Immunol. 93, 140—147 (1964).

SCHMIDT, N. J., E. H. LENNETTE, and M. F. HANAHOE: Microneutralization test for the reoviruses. Application to detection and assay of antibodies in sera of laboratory animals. Proc. Soc. exp. Biol. (N.Y.) 121, 1268—1275 (1966).

SCHNEIDER, I. R., T. O. DIENER, and R. S. SAFFERMAN: Blue-green algal virus LPP-1: Purification and partial characterization. Science 144, 1127—1130 (1964).

SELBY, C. C., C. E. GREY, S. LICHTENBERG, C. FRIEND, A. E. MOORE, and J. J. BIESELE: Submicroscopic cytoplasmic particles occasionally found in the Ehrlich mouse ascites tumor. Cancer Res. 14, 790—794 (1954).

SHATKIN, A. J.: Actinomycin and the differential synthesis of reovirus and L cell RNA. Biochem. biophys. Res. Commun. 19, 506—510 (1965a).

SHATKIN, A. J.: Inactivity of purified reovirus RNA as a template for *E. coli* polymerases *in vitro*. Proc. nat. Acad. Sci. (Wash.) 54, 1721—1728 (1965b).

SHATKIN, A. J., and B. RADA: Reovirus-directed RNA synthesis in infected L cells. J. Virol. 1, 24—35 (1967).

SHAVER, D. N., A. L. BARRON, and D. T. KARZON: Cytopathology of human enteric viruses in tissue culture. Amer. J. Path. 34, 943—963 (1958).

SHIKATA, E., and K. MARAMOROSCH: Electron microscopic evidence for the systemic invasion of an insect host by a plant pathogenic virus. Virology 27, 461—475 (1965).

SHIKATA, E., and K. MARAMOROSCH: An electron microscope study of plant neoplasia induced by wound tumor virus. J. nat. Cancer Inst. 36, 97—116 (1966).

SILAGI, S.: Metabolism of 1-β-d-arabinofuranosylcytosine in L cells. Cancer Res. 25, 1446—1453 (1965).

SIMPSON, D. I. H., A. J. HADDOW, J. P. WOODALL, M. C. WILLIAMS, and T. M. BELL: Attempts to transmit reovirus type 3 by the bite of *Aedes (Stegomyia) aegypti* Linnaeus. E. Afr. med. J. 42, 708—711 (1965).

SMITH, K. O., and J. L. MELNICK: A method for staining virus particles and identifying their nucleic acid type in the electron microscope. Virology 17, 480—490 (1962).

SPENDLOVE, R. S., E. H. LENNETTE, J. N. CHIN, and C. O. KNIGHT: Effect of antimitotic agents on intracellular reovirus antigen. Cancer Res. 24, 1826—1833 (1964).

SPENDLOVE, R. S., E. H. LENNETTE, and A. C. JOHN: The role of the mitotic apparatus in the intracellular location of reovirus antigen. J. Immunol. 90, 554—560 (1963).

SPENDLOVE, R. S., E. H. LENNETTE, C. O. KNIGHT, and J. N. CHIN: Development of viral antigen and infectious virus in HeLa cells infected with reovirus. J. Immunol. 90, 548—553 (1963).

SPENDLOVE, R. S., E. H. LENNETTE, C. O. KNIGHT, and J. N. CHIN: Production in FL cells of infectious and potentially infectious reovirus. J. Bact. 92, 1036—1040 (1966).

SPENDLOVE, R. S., and F. L. SCHAFFER: Enzymatic enhancement of infectivity of reovirus. J. Bact. 89, 597—602 (1965).

STANLEY, N. F.: Relationship of hepatoencephalomyelitis virus and reoviruses. Nature (Lond.) 189, 687 (1961a).

STANLEY, N. F.: Reovirus — An ubiquitous orphan. Med. J. Aust. 2, 815—818 (1961b).

STANLEY, N. F.: The aetiology and pathogenesis of BURKITT's African lymphoma. Lancet **1**, 961—962 (1966a).

STANLEY, N. F.: Virus induction of autoimmune disease and neoplasia. Lancet **II**, 589—590 (1966b).

STANLEY, N. F., D. C. DORMAN, and J. PONSFORD: Studies on the pathogenesis of a hitherto undescribed virus (hepato-encephalomyelitis) producing unusual symptoms in suckling mice. Aust. J. exp. Biol. med. Sci. **31**, 147—159 (1953).

STANLEY, N. F., D. C. DORMAN, and J. PONSFORD: Studies on the hepato-encephalo-myelitis virus (HEV). Aust. J. exp. Biol. med. Sci. **32**, 543—561 (1954).

STANLEY, N. F., and P. J. LEAK: The serologic epidemiology of reovirus infection with special reference to the Rottnest island quokka *(Setonix brachyurus)*. Amer. J. Hyg. **78**, 82—88 (1963).

STANLEY, N. F., P. J. LEAK, G. M. GRIEVE, and D. PERRET: The ecology and epidemiology of reovirus. Aust. J. exp. Biol. med. Sci. **42**, 373—384 (1964).

STANLEY, N. F., P. J. LEAK, M. N.-I. WALTERS, and R. A. JOSKE: Murine infection with reovirus: II. The chronic disease following reovirus type 3 infection. Brit. J. exp. Path. **45**, 142—149 (1964).

STANLEY, N. F., and M. N.-I. WALTERS: Virus induction of autoimmune disease and neoplasia. Lancet **I**, 962—963 (1966).

STANLEY, N. F., M. N.-I. WALTERS, P. J. LEAK, and D. KEAST: The association of murine lymphoma with reovirus type 3 infection. Proc. Soc. exp. Biol. (N.Y.) **121**, 90—93 (1966).

STREISSLE, G., and K. MARAMOROSCH: Similarities between wound-tumor virus and the human-pathogenic reoviruses. Phytopathology **53**, 891 (1963a).

STREISSLE, G., and K. MARAMOROSCH: Reovirus and wound-tumor virus: Serological cross reactivity. Science **140**, 996—997 (1963b).

STRUTSOVSKAYA, A. L., L. YA. ZAKSTELSKAYA, L. V. FEKLISOVA, and A. USMAN-KHODZHAEV: Clinical course of reovirus infection in children. Pediatria **44**, 8—12 (1965). (In Russian.)

STUDDERT, M. J.: Sensitivity of bluetongue virus to ether and sodium deoxycholate. Proc. Soc. exp. Biol. (N.Y.) **118**, 1006—1009 (1965).

STUDDERT, M. J., J. PANGBORN, and R. B. ADDISON: Bluetongue virus structure. Virology **29**, 509—511 (1966).

TAYLOR-ROBINSON, D.: Respiratory virus antibodies in human sera from different regions of the world. Bull. Wld Hlth Org. **32**, 833—847 (1965).

THOMAS, J.-A., et E. DELAIN: Organisation et structure icosaédrique du virus associé à la cellule du carcinome ascitique Krebs 2. C. R. Acad. Sci. (Paris) **261**, 2985—2988 (1965).

THOMAS, J.-A., et E. DELAIN: Développement *in vitro* du réovirus associé à la souche cancéreuse H 22 b; évolution des structures cytoplasmiques en fibres et en tubules. C. R. Acad. Sci. (Paris) **262**, 1028—1031 (1966a).

THOMAS, J.-A., et E. DELAIN: Mise en évidence d'infrastructures ribonucléo-protéiques dans des tubules cytoplasmiques (souche cancéreuse H 22 b avec réo-virus associé). C. R. Acad. Sci. (Paris) **262**, 2255—2258 (1966b).

THOMAS, J.-A., D. DELAIN-VALLET, E. DELAIN et E. HOLLANDE: Isolement et culture du réovirus associé au carcinome ascitique Krebs 2 de la souris: étude du cycle de ce virus, comparativement *in vivo* et *in vitro*, dans une souche de cancer (H 22 b) provoquée chez le hamster. C. R. Acad. Sci. (Paris) **261**, 5721—5724 (1965).

TILLOTSON, J. R., and A. M. LERNER: Isolation of reovirus type 3 from postmortem tissues of a child with a nonbacterial pneumonia. Clin. Res. **14**, 344 (1966).

TOMITA, K.-I., and A. RICH: X-ray diffraction investigations of complementary RNA. Nature (Lond.) **201**, 1160—1163 (1964).

TOTH, M., and A. HONTY: Age-incidence of haemagglutination-inhibiting antibodies to reovirus types 1, 2 and 3. Acta microbiol. Acad. Sci. hung. **13**, 119—126 (1966).

TOURNIER, P., et M. PLISSIER: Le développement intracellulaire du réovirus. Observé au microscope électronique. Presse méd. **68**, 683—688 (1960).

TRAINOR, P. D., S. B. MOHANTY, and F. M. HETRICK: Experimental infection of calves with reovirus type 1. Amer. J. Epidem. **83**, 217—223 (1966).

TURPIN, R., B. CAILLE, F. BRICOUT, J. LAFOURCADE, J. CRUVEILLER, A. KESSELER et C. JOLY: Érythème polymorphe et infection à réovirus. Ann. Pédiat. (Paris) **12**, 36—42 (1965).

USMANKHODZHAYEV, A., L. YA. ZAKSTELSKAYA: Stability of reovirus haemagglu-tinins. Acta virol. **8**, 84—87 (1964).

VAN TONGEREN, H. A. E.: A familial infection with hepato-encephalomyelitis virus in the Netherlands. Study on some properties of the infective agent. Arch. ges. Virusforsch. **7**, 429—448 (1957).

VASQUEZ, C., and P. TOURNIER: The morphology of reovirus. Virology **17**, 503—510 (1962).

VASQUEZ, C., and P. TOURNIER: New interpretation of the reovirus structure. Virology **24**, 128—130 (1964).

WALLIS, C., and J. L. MELNICK: Cationic stabilization — A new property of entero-viruses. Virology **16**, 504—505 (1962).

WALLIS, C., and J. L. MELNICK: Irreversible photosensitization of viruses. Virology **23**, 520—527 (1964).

WALLIS, C., J. L. MELNICK, and M. BIANCHI: Factors influencing enterovirus and reovirus growth and plaque formation. Tex. Rep. Biol. Med. **20**, 693—702 (1962).

WALLIS, C., J. L. MELNICK, and F. RAPP: Effects of pancreatin on the growth of reovirus. J. Bact. **92**, 155—160 (1966).

WALLIS, C., K. O. SMITH, and J. L. MELNICK: Reovirus activation by heating and inactivation by cooling in MgCl₂ solutions. Virology **22**, 608—619 (1964).

WALTERS, M. N.-I., R. A. JOSKE, P. J. LEAK, and N. F. STANLEY: Murine infection with reovirus: I. Pathology of the acute phase. Brit. J. exp. Path. **44**, 427—436 (1963).

WALTERS, M. N.-I., P. J. LEAK, R. A. JOSKE, N. F. STANLEY, and D. H. PERRET: Murine infection with reovirus. III. Pathology of infection with types 1 and 2. Brit. J. exp. Path. **46**, 200—212 (1965).

WENNER, H. A., and T. D. Y. CHIN: Discussion in Cellular Biology, Nucleic Acids, and Viruses. Spec. Publ. N.Y. Acad. Sci. **5**, 384—387 (1957).

ZALAN, E., and N. A. LABZOFFSKY: Interference between proflavine treated reovirus and related and unrelated viruses. Arch. ges. Virusforsch. **15**, 200—209 (1965).

ZALAN, E., W. D. LEERS, and N. A. LABZOFFSKY: Occurrence of reovirus infection in Ontario. Canad. med. Ass. J. **87**, 714—715 (1962).

ZALAN, E., J. LESIAK, and N. A. LABZOFFSKY: The effect of proflavine on the hem-agglutinating activity of reo- and ECHO viruses. Canad. J. Microbiol. **8**, 181—187 (1962).